T0150083

VERONICA ANDERSON, MD

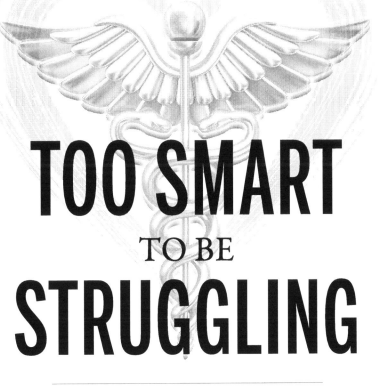

TOO SMART
TO BE
STRUGGLING

The Guide for Over-Scheduled
Doctors to Find **HAPPINESS**
(And Make **MORE MONEY**, Too)

TOO SMART TO BE STRUGGLING
The Guide for Over-Scheduled Doctors to Find Happiness
(And Make More Money, Too)

Difference Press, Washington, D.C., USA

© Dr. Veronica Anderson, 2020

ISBN: 978-1-68309-272-8

Cover Design: Jennifer Stimson
Interior Book Design: Anna Zubrytska
Editing: Cory Hott
Author Photo Credit: Stacey Lievens Green

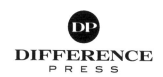

DIFFERENCE
P R E S S

To my mother and father who carried the vision of me as a doctor and healer from when I was still an angel in heaven until now.

ADVANCE PRAISE

"Dr. Veronica's book is a timely resource for all women physicians who have reached a plateau in their career. She creates a plan to conquer burnout and maximize your potential! I encourage anyone who feels like they want more from their job to read it."

~ Helen M Blake, MD, President-Elect, Women Innovators in Pain Medicine, Author of Fulfilled: How to Thrive as a Female Physician

Burnout is pandemic among medical professionals. As a result, practitioners' health, their life satisfaction, and the quality of care they provide are on the decline. Dr. Veronica Anderson shatters the stereotype that success must come with struggle, and lays out a road map for creating a joyful, prosperous, and healthy life. This is a must-read for physicians. And if you're thinking right now, "I'm too busy to read a book," sounds like you're holding a solution in your hands.

-Dr. Valerie Rein, psychologist, author of "Patriarchy Stress Disorder: The Invisible Inner Barrier to Women's Happiness and Fulfillment. "Creator of the only science-backed system for helping women achieve their ultimate success and happiness. www.drvalerie.com

This is an heroic book. Absolutely outside the box. Conventional, allopathic doctors [MDs/DOs] are in a whole lot of hurt. As late

as 20 years ago they were on a societal pedestal. With the advent of the Internet, big Medi-business, the growth of Medicare and dominance of insurance companies, doctors are now commoditized and too often reduced to turnstile medicine. This has resulted in a massive decline in societal and self-perceived "value." The result is practicing their art of medicine against very strong headwinds, and hence a very much higher likelihood of burnout. Dr. Anderson had personal experience with this state. Her book offers an amazing prescription to help with the professional burnout syndrome. Her perspectives and solutions are beyond conventional cognitive behavioral therapy. As an MD, she herself is beyond convention. I only hope that conventional physicians, or other health professionals, experiencing or concerned about their own burnout, can step outside their normal boxes to avail themselves of Dr. Anderson's prescriptions. I'm certain they would be helped. Like her, I too, about two decades ago, decided to step outside the conventional medical box and follow my internal compass. I can't tell you how much happier and more satisfied I am professionally. I can also tell you that my patients appreciate and are the recipients of this form of heartfelt medicine.

-William Pawluk, MD, MSc. Author of "Power Tools for Health: how pulsed magnetic fields [PEMFs] help you." Host: Pain Solution Summit; PainSolutionSummit.com. drpawluk.com

"This book gives health care professionals practical guidance on how to overcome career anxiety, burnout, and frustration of practicing medicine. It feels like Dr. Veronica is right there cheering you on."

—Steven Masley, MD, FAHA, FACN, FAAFP, CNS, author of The Mediterranean Method."

The practice of medicine continues to evolve but so do you as a physician and a human being. Considering new options and changing your course during your career is a complicated and often lonely experience. This book may help you find the tools and support you need to take a new path.

-Mary Clifton, M.D., America's Telemedicine Doctor,

CBD and Cannabis Expert

Since I started this new venture, I have read many entrepreneurship books, but Dr. Anderson really dug into the problems we as physicians face specifically, including our entrenched way of being that we start conditioning in medical school. Some of what she says shook up my very sense of who I am as a physician. Some of this made me question my reality, but it uncovered important blind spots, and was the necessary shake I needed to be able to press forward. I recommend this book to any physician who is considering breaking free from what their original plan was.

~ Leah Houston, MD, Emergency Physician, HPEC CEO

The medical system is broken, and so are the doctors. Dr. Veronica Anderson has journeyed from passionate healthcare provider to disillusioned, retired physician. Unlike most doctors, though, she discovered a way to reinvent herself AND the healthcare system she works with so that it serves both doctor and patient. Dr. Anderson brings together the heart of a healer and the acumen of a successful businesswoman. She shows physicians who have abandoned their dreams how to re-purpose years of experience into work that sparks their heart and rekindles the joy in their lives.

This book is a rare gem: a wise-woman-physician's cure for burnout, and a guide for fulfilling the dream that propelled you to medical school in the first place.

-Judith Boice, ND, LAc, FABNO, author of The Green Medicine
Chest and Soul Medicine.

Every unhappy doctor needs to reschedule a bunch of patients today and read this book! The health of the medical field would be enormously transformed if this was required reading for maintaining a medical license. Learn from Dr. Veronica's struggle, it's time to get real and triage your stressed filled life STAT!"

-Lisa Cherney, Host of Get F***ing Real Podcast

"The step-by-step process that Dr. Anderson provides you in this book is worth its weight in gold! Knowing how to transition from being ready to quit medicine to enjoying your career again is priceless. This book has straightforward strategies that anyone can use to overcome the key fears associated with making this transition. Excellent job Dr. Anderson!" –

-Evan H. Hirsch, MD, best-selling author and creator of
the Fix Your Fatigue Program

"A radical look at the unacknowledged challenges that medical doctors face, Too Smart to Be Struggling sheds light on a culture in desperate need of revitalization. Through her own story of being a successful ophthalmologist who burned out under the inhuman strain that many doctors face, Dr Veronica shares her path to the other side. The resilience and financial abundance she discovered outside of the traditional medical system is readily available to everyone. With trailblazing clarity, Dr. Veronica shows the way to freedom from the medical grind to true gratification in your

work. *Groundbreaking information that will make you stop and reevaluate the spell that has captured so many of our brightest minds and biggest hearts.*"

-Robin Winn, LMFT, international bestselling author of *Understanding Your Clients through Human Design.*

"*It's hard not to see yourself in this book if you've poured your blood, sweat and tears into the long journey of pursuing medicine for your career. It's comforting to know you're not alone AND that Dr. Veronica gives you a roadmap so you don't have to go it alone either.*"

-Dr. Kiera Barr, Author *"The Skin Whisperer: A Dermatologist Reveals How to Look Younger, Radiate Beauty and Create the Life you Crave",* www.drkeirabarr.com

Physician burnout is real and largely a taboo to speak about for fear of increased scrutiny. I can never thank Dr. Veronica enough for writing this book. She shares unapologetically how burnout affected her personal and professional life and her personal decision to walk away from a successful ophthalmology practice with over 11,000 patients to search for her true calling. After doing her own work, she has emerged as a beacon of light and courage willing to share with her colleagues a protocol to help them gain clarity surrounding not only their career goals but their life goals. Do not just read this book, implement her strategies.

-Dr. Eno Nsima-Obot, Functional medicine consultant, speaker, and award-winning author

"*Dr. Veronica shows us the fundamental missing link in the dream of the perfect medical career and presents a clear program for leaving behind the burnout and frustration so many doctors* are feeling these days. Fantastic and straightforward. Highly recommend even if you're not facing burnout (yet!)"

-Jane Guyn PhD, Relationship coach and author of the #1 Amazon Bestseller "Too Busy to Get Busy"

Dr. Veronica shares powerful secrets for doctors and professionals who suffer from burn out, fatigue and depression. Award winning!

-Louise Swartswalter,ND- Beautiful Brain Expert

I work with burnt out people every day - I call it Total Body Meltdown. Successful treatment incorporates the nutrient building blocks (especially magnesium) for our cells that translates into a solid structure that leads to energetic functioning of the body. I feel that it's with a strong body that the mental, emotional, and spiritual that Dr. Veronica covers so well, will fall into place. Incorporating those nutrients in their practice, patients would become healthier and praise their doctors instead of blaming them, which would lessen one major factor that does cause doctor burnout.

~ Carolyn F. A. Dean MD ND, author of The Magnesium Miracle (2017)

This must-read book shines the light on the barb-wired walls of the dark institution of modern healthcare, and provides the inspiration and blueprint to plan your escape, so you can live life and practice medicine on your terms.

-Alex Lubarsky, CEO Health Media Group, Inc Author: The Art of Selling The Art of Healing

Dr. Veronica's depth of knowledge and experience makes her the perfect person to write this much needed book! The face of health *care is changing and we need to change with it. I highly recommend this book to every health care professional who's ready to make a change for the better!*

-Lisa Kafer, Healthy Lifestyle coach & author of "The Layman's Guide to a Healthier You", www.cleanfoodcleanyou.com

Dr. Veronica is a rare combination of being a giver and healer in her capacity as physician and intuitive, while also being a successful entrepreneur. Her attitude towards abundance and self care is an example for all physicians. Based on my career working with many 1000s of clients on the severe end of burnout and chronic fatigue, and my experience in business as a chartered accountant and health entrepreneur, I can confirm her advice is solid, practical, and if you can implement it, will be sure to change your life forever. Physicians deserve to have a happy, abundant and fulfilling life – Dr Veronica can show you how!

-Niki Gratrix, Dip ION NANP The Abundant Energy Expert. Functional Health and Transformation Coach, host of The Abundant Energy Summit www.nikigratrix.com

"I find anyone practicing and serving others with the wide and varied modalities of health and wellness is a great hope for humanity at large. The work Dr. Veronica is doing will go far beyond the natural world to help heal self, community and the world. Seek her out, work with her and move from survival to 'THRIVAL'. Many, many blessings"

-Richard Dugan, Host: Tell Me Your Story. Author: Choices-5 Steps for Life

"After having the honor and pleasure of meeting Dr Veronica on my show, I was instantly inspired by her energy, information, and wisdom. Her book "Too Smart to be Struggling" is absolutely

amazing! It is a must read. Thank you, Veronica, for this gift to all of us."

-Paula Neva Vail, author of "Why am I so Happy", Host of "Choices: Finding your Joy", and founder of www.wellnessinspired.com

I am really happy that Dr. Anderson has written this book. The way things are set up for doctors currently is not working for them or their patients (Us!), and I see that in the number of doctors who have given up trying to work within the system, and struck out on their own. And this is the best case scenario! I worry that we are losing even more good doctors who just leave and move onto other work, never having realized their potential to truly contribute to the health and wellbeing of thousands of people. I hope this book becomes part of the movement for the change that is so needed in our healthcare system.

-Katherine Miller, Executive Health & Energy Coach, Menopause Guide

Master Plant-Powered Chef, Mbodiedwomen.com

Radiant KickAss Women's Club

TABLE OF CONTENTS

Chapter 1

SHOULD I QUIT MEDICINE?

Forty-four percent of physicians are burned out.

Eleven percent are colloquially depressed, and four percent are clinically depressed.

Forty-nine percent of internal medicine physicians suffer from burnout.

Forty-eight percent of emergency medicine physicians and forty percent of emergency medicine and family physicians are burnt out. The list goes on and on and on.

Fifty percent of female physicians and thirty-nine percent of male physicians suffer from burnout.

What is contributing to this burnout?

I'm sure you can list the reasons off the top of your head, just like I can.

Reasons like too many tasks, such as charting and filling out patient paperwork (or, should I say, those electronic medical records); spending too many hours at work; the increasing computerization of the practice with electronic health records; a lack of respect from administrators, employers, colleagues, staff, and even patients; and insufficient compensation and reimbursements.

Add to that, the high debt that was taken out to get to this point in your career, the lack of autonomy and control, government regulations, feeling like a cog in a wheel, the emphasis on profits over patients, and on and on and on.

You see your perfect career, what you dreamed of at night and thought about when you were a kid, and it's nothing like that now. Those long hours have taken a toll on not just you, but your family too.

You've missed important birthdays, you've missed weddings, you've missed vacations, you've missed a part of your youth. Guess what? More and more of us are working within organizations. Those organizations are driving us hard.

I liken it to sharecropping. You work hard with someone else calling the shots. Sometimes you get paid. Other times you don't. You work a lot of hours so that the hourly wages end up way below minimum wage. Work hours are long. You are penalized for resting, eating, and peeing. I felt like a slave a lot of days, except intermittently and unpredictably after begging and pleading with either insurance companies or patients, you get some money. It wasn't me directly begging and pleading. I had a staff to do that, but I am sure you get what I mean. Those insurance companies would do everything to pay you very low or not at all. "Not a covered service" would be the explanation on the claim denial. Of course, you had already done the work, seen the patient, helped them get better. Then the insurance givers you the head fake. You are pretty sure that what you are doing is covered. Why wouldn't it be? The patient is clearly sick. But somehow, the service you provided isn't covered. My staff would call and fight for the money, but if they didn't, there were the dreaded words at the bottom of the claim with the asterisk, "Patient not responsible. Do not bill." The Plantation called Maison Medicine.

Here are some of the words my colleagues have shared to show how burnout has affected them.

"I dread coming to work. I find myself being short in dealing with staff and patients."

"I'm having medical problems as a result of having recurrent miscarriages and drinking more and more, and have become less active."

"My relationships have withered. My family is frustrated. We rarely make plans to do anything socially, as they are likely to be canceled."

These are words from the Medscape National Physician Burnout, Depression, and Suicide Report of 2019.

We doctors have been attempting to deal with our burnout on our own and in isolation. Because, you know, we all have trouble asking for help.

What do we do? We've been exercising. We've been talking to our friends. But one of the most important issue is, we've been isolating ourselves from others. Some other things I've been seeing:

We've turned to abuse of alcohol and drugs. One of my good friends from medical school lost his license due to alcohol abuse. Nineteen of us are dealing with our burnout by binge eating.

Why do we need to get this problem fixed?

Well, we need to get the joy back in life because everyone deserves joy, even those of us who are doctors and caregivers. We work every day to help give other people their joy.

But on the other side, the issues we have been having in our profession with burnout, anxiety, and depression are affecting how we are caring for our patients.

Thirty-five percent of us are saying that we get exasperated easily with our patients, and twenty-six percent of us are less motivated to be careful when taking care of patient notes. We're expressing frustration in front of patients and making errors that we would not normally make.

These errors can lead to devastating effects in the lives of our patients, as well as devastating long-term effects on our lives as we deal with lawsuits and public relations nightmares.

Physician suicide rates are some of the highest in the country.

Did you know that PTSD is higher in doctors than it is in veterans who've been in a war?

Yet, few of us seek help for our burnout and depression.

When surveyed in the Medscape 2019 report, sixty-four percent of physicians said that we didn't plan to seek professional help. Thirteen percent responded that they had sought professional help in the past and another sixteen percent said that they are seeking professional help or plan to seek professional help.

What does this mean? My interpretation of this data is that a large portion of physicians have decided that we're going to go through these issues on our own.

When you go to conferences, you can see doctors walking around like zombies. You can see the misery on their faces.

Everybody's acting like everything is okay, but the energy in the room is low and dark.

Why don't we seek help if we feel like that? Maybe we feel the symptoms are not severe enough, or that we can deal with it without help from a professional. Or that we're too busy.

But there's another factor.

We don't want to risk that this trouble we're having may be disclosed.

Given that many of us are feeling bad, we want to feel better, and we'd love to have a solution, whether it means leaving medicine or staying.

How are we going to work this out?

When I was going through it, I wished there was a road map, a blueprint, a guide, something. But you know, with the demands of my work, running a practice with all the people and employees under me, all the paperwork that needed to be done, plus my family responsibility with a husband and three young kids, I just didn't have time to get it all figured out.

I wanted somebody to point me to the way.

But I didn't even have time to figure out where to go look.

To show you, step by step, how to take back control of your life – how to reclaim meaning and happiness, and actually, to give yourself a raise or get a raise.

You have to start somewhere. Here it is. I want to make it easy for you, one-stop shopping. I don't want you to have to run around, because you don't have time to run around. In fact, you probably have to run away now to go do something else.

I promise you're going to have answers. Some, in fact, before the end of the book. I bet you'll have made a decision about the best step or best path forward for you, whether it be to stay where you are, but with new joy and vigor and a new way of practicing medicine, or move to a new career altogether.

The important part is that you figure out what you're supposed to do at this point in life and how to do it. I'm going to give you some tips and tools in each step to get it figured out quickly.

The first thing you have to do is make the commitment to yourself that you're going to do things differently. It's so cliché, but so true what Einstein said about the definition of insanity: doing the same thing over and over and expecting a different result. But we do the same thing over and over because we see no other options. My wish for you is that you leave behind the insanity of feeling bad, the insanity of being out of control, the insanity of exhaustion, the insanity of being overworked and overwhelmed, the insanity of being under-compensated.

By the end of this book, you'll be able to answer the question, "Should I quit medicine?" and, whether the answer is yes or no, you'll know precisely what your next move is and how to do it.

Chapter 2

YOU KNOW THE TROUBLE I'VE SEEN

I know. I've been there, just like you.

I had those days of feeling so miserable and dejected, and I couldn't figure out how my dream had fallen apart.

I came to a crossroads trying to figure out if I should quit medicine.

I wanted to be a doctor since I was four years old, and I was excited about medicine. I worked hard in college, went through medical school, and was excited on the day I walked across that stage, with those three stripes on my sleeves, to receive my medical diploma.

But what happened?

From my time in college, through starting my practice, and as my practice was going on, the landscape of the health care system in America changed. The policy changed. Demands changed. Most of all, reimbursements decreased.

I worked harder and harder just to stay afloat. it seemed like every day, nobody appreciated what I did for them.

I just wanted out. Or, at least, I wanted to go back to the way I thought it should be.

I thought, is there something else I can do besides medicine? Who should I talk to? How do I get this all figured out?

I needed some answers. Is there a book about this, or a study I can read? Or, at least, a case study?

One day, I simply couldn't take it anymore. I was depressed. Later on, I found out I had what's called physician burnout. I couldn't stand going to work every day.

In fact, I couldn't even get to my office or the operating room on time. I was reprimanded for being late to the operating room because I felt so miserable.

Let's break down what's going on.

I'm sure you're going to.

I dreamed of being a doctor. Even back when I was a four-year-old girl, I said to my mother in the kitchen, "Hey, Mom, I like helping people. I want to be a nurse." My mother said to me, "Roni, you're bright, so be a doctor. You'll have more control."

I can hear in my mind the voice of Louis Armstrong right about now single the spiritual.

> *"Nobody knows the trouble I've seen.*
> *Nobody knows my sorrow.*
> *Nobody knows the trouble I've seen."*

Oh boy, was my mother so wrong. I want you to know about my mother. She has always been a wise and reliable confidante and able to see situations for what they are. She has provided such invaluable advice in my life. There's no way she could have predicted how my conventional medical career was going to turn out. I remember being in the hospital operating room as an attending ophthalmologist during my time in practice, and the nurses who were the administrators were telling me what to do. The doctors were not in control of anything. Doctors are the cogs in the wheel and nothing more.

You know how there are moments in your life where you start to question everything? Well, that's what happened.

I graduated from Princeton. Like you, being an over-achiever, I was admitted into eight medical schools.

I decided to go to medical school in New Jersey because I got a scholarship. I was so happy to have that scholarship. I feel blessed to have been given money, so I wouldn't have much debt when I graduated.

When I went to school, it wasn't so bad. Actually, I could just memorize everything. It was great. I was lucky enough to have that strong memory, but also to go through the clinical rotations and be able to diagnose easily.

I graduated with honors.

I went on to my residency in internal medicine, working 85- to 100-hour weeks.

Then, five days before medical school graduation, I had my first child. I was pregnant all through my third and my fourth year of medical school. I even went to ophthalmology residency interviews pregnant, hiding my pregnancy because I knew that if anyone knew I was pregnant, I was not going to get a position.

As an intern, I had an infant. Being so tired from working those 85-100-hour weeks meant that I neglected to put in my diaphragm for contraception. Thus, baby number two was cooking in the oven. I was an intern running around floors, being in this CCU and that ICU running codes, noisy, the whole nine yards. One day, on-call at Princeton Medical Center, I went into preterm labor at thirty-two weeks.

When I was in the hospital in preterm labor, I called my ophthalmology residency program, which I was due to start on July 1. My baby was due in mid-July.

The residency director was a woman. When I told her this, she said, "Oh, it's not a good time to have a baby."

What do you think I could do? I was already pregnant. The female residency director saying to me "It's not a good time to have a baby" is the kind of snark you put up with when you go into medicine.

I finally went into labor again at thirty-six weeks. One day, less than twenty-four hours after the medicine to stop labor was discontinued.

The baby's heartrate was going into the decelerations and slowing down dangerously. The doctor sat by me for hours, with her hands gripping the edge of her chair, trying to decide whether she should let me continue laboring or take me to the operating room for a Caesarean section. Finally, I delivered my baby. The umbilical cord was wrapped around his neck three times. Luckily, the cord was taken from around his neck, the delivery was done, and I had my second healthy baby boy – thirteen months after my first child was born and thirteen days before my residency would be gone.

I did go into my ophthalmology residency, thirteen days postpartum, with a thirteen-month-old toddler and a thirteen-day-old infant at home.

You know the demands – I don't have to tell you about it. But then, I decided I was going to do a fellowship. I did a fellowship and interviewed for several jobs, and later on, decided, "You know what, I'm going to start a practice." I went out and started my practice, building it from patient zero up to digits in the thousands.

Being an eye surgeon meant that I could have cash-producing, non-insurance services in my practice. Now luckily, I've always liked business and marketing. I give talks around town, was written about in newspaper articles, and appeared on many radio interviews. I built a thriving, full-service eye care practice.

Along the way, some crappy things happened. First of all, there are the jerky patients who complain they have to wait too long.

I loved most of my patients, but the days when those jerky patients came in just made life miserable, especially when I'm running around the office and haven't had anything to eat all day, including lunch. It's three o'clock, and I haven't even peed.

As I'm going along in my practice, my patients love me and I love them, but I hate the business of medicine, even though I had a practice that made cash flow decently. I was making almost a million dollars a year, and working kind of part-time-ish because I still had a husband and two kids to take care of, and I wanted to be around them sometime. But it was still me, taking calls and missing birthday parties and events, because, of course, you always get called when there's something important that you want to do in your life, and you can't say no when you're the first in line to go to the emergency room.

I worked with the Cancer Institute in New Jersey, helping them do studies and seeing patients on the inpatient list with eye problems due to their cancers and the complications of cancer treatments.

I went into ophthalmology so that I wouldn't have to see people die. I saw a lot of people die, and it was a little depressing some days. What was even more depressing was the very unpredictable revenue coming into my practice. Some weeks it was quite a lot and others it was paltry. Even though I'm telling you how much money I was able to make, there were months where my bank account would drain down to zero because the insurance companies weren't paying, even though I had significant receivables with them. I had to dip into my line of credit to pay my employees, and I didn't pay myself.

Now, if you're employed by a hospital, you don't necessarily know these particular stresses, but I'm sure you've heard them from your private practice friends. You think that those of us in those Rolls Royce specialties like ophthalmology never have cash flow problems, but we do. I was upset because I realized that it was getting worse every year. Reimbursements were going down, so I had to see more patients, and you know how that works. I was drained. I was at home, being the runner back and forth to take my husband to the train station, taking care of my kids. I even homeschooled my kids one year while working in my office.

Why did I do this? Because I'm just like you. I'm an overachiever and a perfectionist, and that meant that I wanted to be a perfect wife, a perfect mother, and a perfect doctor too.

Let me tell you about when I was a Sunday school teacher, because this will become relevant as I guide you through the process.

My then-husband and I taught a financial course on how to manage finances, according to biblical principles. It was one of the most popular Sunday school classes, and I still have people today who, when they run into me, tell me how much that course changed their lives. I am super happy about that. Because of the double-digit thousands of patients I had in my practice, it was rare for people to come up to me and tell me that my work as a doctor was important to them and it changed their life. You see, being a doctor can be thankless a lot of days.

Sometimes, being appreciated is more than the money. But you know what, after you've worked 100-hour weeks, graduated with honors, and neglected your family, you expect to get paid. You don't expect the struggle, and you don't expect some months to not have enough money in the bank to be able to pay yourself, even though you're doing all the work. Suddenly, up the line comes some seriously demoralizing lawsuits.

The first lawsuit had nothing to do with my medical care.

A patient and his family I took care of for several years had Oxford insurance.

I had seen them and taken care of them. Oxford Insurance would not pay.

And the reason they wouldn't pay is because this family didn't give the insurance company all the information they asked for. What did that mean? They didn't pay me.

Well, we billed the patient, because they said they weren't paying. We were well within our rights to bill the patient, even according to Oxford insurance.

This man was a businessman and wanted to buy a restaurant. We sent this to our collection agency, and the collection agent sent a nice letter to them. We would send out a letter that said, "You owe us this amount of money. We ask that you pay this within thirty days or contact our office to make arrangements. If you don't make arrangements, you're not going to hear from us again about this, we're simply going to report it to the credit bureau." Now this was a pleasant letter. most people would call up and they would pay their bills, or they would speak with their insurance company and make them pay the bill, or they would make payment arrangements. But not this gentleman.

He decided he was going to sue me. The reason that he sued me was because, when he applied for credit when he was opening a restaurant, he got a higher interest rate.

I contacted my lawyer.

My lawyer said, "You are absolutely right. You would win this case, but it will cost you more to pay me and be out of your office with this than to just settle the case. Offer him a little bit of money and settle the case." So that's what we did.

Now this is symbolic of how it goes in medicine.

I was right. But I had to pay.

Lawsuit number two.

I was a glaucoma specialist. I took care of difficult patients.

Mr. V. had a hard-to-control glaucoma.

I had done several lasers on him and a previous operation. Then, we had to go to the operating room again.

As with all my patients, I was safe, rather than sorry. I ordered preoperative lab testing.

There were a few abnormalities noted by me on his blood test. There was this little spot on one rib found on his chest X-ray.

These small abnormalities did not put him at risk, so I didn't need to cancel his surgery, which was to be done under local anesthesia. I simply called up and alerted his primary care doctor that I sent him to her for an evaluation, and it was discovered that he had a blood cancer.

Although due to the pre-operative testing I ordered before his glaucoma surgery and my referral to his doctor for a work up of these abnormalities which resulted in the diagnosis and treatment that was likely life-saving, the patient sued for a reason I still cannot fathom. He sued both me and his primary doctors, who did what we were supposed to which was work up and refer to an oncologist.

I remember going to the deposition and the lawyer telling me, "It was the strangest thing. I've never seen a case like this. When I was in to question your patient, he was just so complimentary and nice and smiley and couldn't say enough nice things about you."

The case was eventually dropped – at least, I was dropped from the case. His primary care was dropped from the case. I don't know what happened from the rest of it, but you know how lawsuits go, they can keep you tied up and stressed for at least two years, if not more. Two years after I got the notice that I was being sued, I was dropped from the case because his lawyers did not feel I had done anything that warranted further litigation.

Miss E came to my office as another challenging glaucoma patient.

She had thick glasses. She had lost her vision in one eye years ago.

She had a history of rubella as a child, which meant that she developed cataracts and glaucoma, an exceedingly difficult situation in her good eye. She had previous cataract surgery, without the lens being put in. She was developing another opacity in that eye, and her vision was getting worse.

There was a laser procedure that I could do. But I was concerned. Well, this lady walks in and she says, "I can't see but I'm scared to have anything done, because I'm scared I'm gonna go blind."

I looked at what needed to be done. Yag laser capsulotomy, in which you use the laser to punch a hole into the cloudy lens remnants in the eye so that the patient can regain vision, is an office procedure. I had thousands of these types of lasers and others without ever once having any complications.

As life can go at times, on the lady with one blind eye and another eye that could see but required the procedure, a problem occurs. A big one.

The next day after the laser, on the first post-laser visit, the pressure in her eye was very high, and she could hardly see out of her one good eye.

Now, the interesting part about this all is, as I evaluated her going forward, her vision wasn't returning as it should have. Her eye looked the same as it had before. I couldn't figure out why she couldn't see. I sent her to the neuro-ophthalmologist. He could not figure out why she couldn't see, because her eye looked the same as it had five years before. I sent her to another specialist, a retinal specialist who had seen her previously. He couldn't figure out why she couldn't see, either. I felt like crap. Horrible. A failure even though I had done everything the same as I had thousands of times before this procedure. The lady couldn't read the eye chart. Not even the big E! Yet none of us could tell why she couldn't see or figure out a treatment for her to bring back her vision.

That's the first day I felt like I wanted to go jump off a bridge.

I was doing everything I could to help her, and yet she was unable to see in her only eye.

This is when the full depression hit – the pressures of home combined with the pressures of feeling like crap, because someone had a bad outcome that I couldn't even explain. What are you supposed to do when you are helpless and the doctors you refer to aren't able to help?

I have to point out at this point that I was extremely fortunate to have colleagues who were willing to help and understood that this case was rare and unusual, so they did not talk me down. They simply said to both me and the patient that they could not explain the problem. Unfortunately, there are some physicians that will talk down their colleagues more than is necessary, and this type of behavior among physicians is one of those things that leads many of us to the levels of burnout and depression and suicide.

It's hard for me to tell the story, even now. She did sue – one day before the statute of limitations ran out, the lawsuit papers arrived in my office. By this point in time, I had gotten so depressed that I had walked out of my office six months previously. That left all the other doctors there, and I decided I wasn't returning, although I never told anybody. I quit six months before that. When I came back to check on my office, as I was deciding to leave my practice, the lawsuit papers showed up.

Her lawyer asked me everything in the deposition.

She made me feel as if I should have never even graduated from kindergarten, because I was incompetent at everything in life. Lawyers are the consummate Monday morning quarterback; they know everything about everything even though they have not spent even one day in medical school or taking care of patients with countless complicated medical problems in an ever changing situation. Yet lawyers can be quite gifted at pointing out all the things and reasons you did practically everything wrong in a particular case and the rest of your entire life, too.

My lawyer asked me: "Veronica, would you have done anything different with this patient?" My answer was, "I should have listened to her. Never touched her." Remember, that was only when she said she was going to go blind.

Now, within the lawsuit. I want you to know that the doctor that certified that I could be sued said that, from reading the chart, he could not see that I did something wrong.

But my lawyer recommended that I settle, because the case was too complex to be able to explain to a lay jury, and the patient was pitiful. Although from looking at the case, I was not at fault, it was best for me to settle because it was not certain that we could prove this to a lay jury, who doesn't understand the nuances of medicine.

We settled.

As all this going on, I fell into a deep depression.

I decided I didn't want to be married anymore.

I didn't want to go to church anymore.

I didn't want to be a doctor anymore.

Because if this is how it's going to be, being a practicing physician just is not worth it.

I walked out of my office.

I laid on the ground for many days, surprised that the sun came up, because I felt so depleted.

I questioned every decision I had made in life. My dream was gone.

I found a good psychologist, and I had to go to the psychologist twice a week.

She made me realize that it was worth living because there was a lot of life ahead of me.

I got a divorce.

I feel like it was medicine and working too hard, and expecting everything to be perfect that lead to my dissatisfaction with my marriage and my life in general. Patients and the healthcare system expected me to be perfect. My husband expected me to be a perfect wife and mother, and my church expected me to be that impossible kind of perfect, or risk going into the fire forevermore.

But there's light at the end of the tunnel.

With the help of a good psychologist and therapy plus my personal trainer, Dave S, who would deal with me bursting out in tears in the middle of my training sessions, I got up and began to move on in life.

When I was in my eyecare practice, I was always talking about health and wellness issues with my clients. I decided, "You know what? I'm going to go to Peru on a mission and work in an eye clinic for a little while," which I did.

Then, I'm going to start coaching people on how to be well. I'm going to do some media. I'm going to coach. I'm going to leave behind ophthalmology. I finally just closed the doors of my practice. I hadn't gone back. I had other doctors working for me, but I just completely closed the doors. I began to move on.

Well, during this whole time, I realized even more that I have visions. I realized that I know things about people, and I've always known things about people with no explanation. I would know things about my patients with no explanation. This is why I was such a good clinician, I would know the answer without any data points. Then I would do the questions in an exam to fill in and verify that I had the right answer.

During this time is when I was noticing that I have what is called "clairvoyance." I could see what life is like from looking in my mind at pictures that look like a movie. I'll know about other people, places, and things. I kept my mouth shut for lots of years because I'm a real doctor.

This was during the time when I was keeping my mouth shut. Well, the beauty of life is, as I'm walking along in life, my friend Bonnie says, "I think you should see my psychic." I go visit her psychic. She predicts that I'm going to get married again. This is October of 2010.

This is how life presents itself to me. It's about taking the leap and risks to get something wonderful. This is all happening as I'm starting my coaching and consulting business. I'm frequently appearing on radio shows as a guest and beginning to host a podcast. My business is working (by that I mean cash flowing), and I started doing high ticket consulting to help people transform their health.

I realized that I had gone through this awakening and gotten clear about who I am and clear about the people that I can help. I started marketing directly to those people. One of my first sales was to a couple for $13,000 to do a six-month health transformation coaching and consulting for them.

Life with my new hubby was good. We started an export business. In that export business, I was the face of the business for marketing, because you know I got good at that stuff. I was email marketing, and we were exporting cars, and people all over the world got to know me as the face of American Car Exporters.

Because they saw that I was a doctor, people would send me messages on Skype, on Facebook, and on WhatsApp, and say, "You're a doctor. Can you help me?" All of a sudden, I realized that I knew exactly what was wrong with these people without having seen them or talked to them, but just by getting a text message. I mean, names of diagnosis would pop in my head like "malignant hypertension" written in the sky.

"His mother has heart disease and she's going to go into the hospital. His father is wasting away and is sad that his son won't talk to him."

After this, even when I started my consulting practice, and they would ask me a question about their health and the writing across the sky would appear. Black, bold lettering in the blue sky with a few nimbus clouds. "Acquired Acromegaly," one read. That was the first and only time I have seen that outside a medical textbook. I forgot it even existed, but I knew what test to tell her to go tell her doctor to order. Yes, in my head. Even without seeing people. I would get these Zebra diagnoses. You know most things are horses and every once in a while it's the Zebra or more like the Unicorn. This is largely how things came to me when I was in my medical practice.

People just thought I was wonderfully brilliant, and yes. But you know, to be book-smart and take a test is not the same as being a brilliant clinician, and I could diagnose all kinds of things outside of my specialty, because I would get the download. I tell you this because, when I developed the courage to fully embrace my woo woo gifts and talents, it became one of the most important ways that I help people with their health and other things in their life and business.

Telling the story about the writing in the sky is perilous because there are groups of doctors who think only they are uniquely qualified to tell people what's wrong after they do it the way laid out by somebody like the American Board of This or The Society of That or the Medical Licensing Board of the State of Whatever of the Fifty States You Want to Drop In Here. In the U.S. of A., never do I give a diagnosis that appears in the ICD. I have to figure out all the ways around it so colleagues won't be crappy towards me. Clients are happy I exist and use whatever I can to help them through their woes. Doctors on the other hand, especially anyone with an MD, seem to think they have to stamp out anything they have approved in all in the name of "protecting the public." Sickening and killing people accidentally with pharmaceuticals? Completely acceptable. Helping people heal with means that has no side effects but isn't on PubMed? Absolutely questionable.

Thus, I began my career as a Medical Intuitive, but it was not so easy, because I was afraid of you – my medical colleagues – talking about me.

Until I had a big injury.

I didn't want to embrace this.

Let me tell you about one big turning point.

I was running and training for a 10k. I leave my apartment at around noon on March 2, 2013 to take a run (I am not an elite athlete, so some would smirk when I call what I do running). I didn't want to go running that day, but I said "I gotta do a training run." As I go down the street on Fifth Avenue, and I run past the Metropolitan Museum of Art, I trip and fall on 76th Street. I can't catch myself and into the middle of the street I fall, oh my god, I have so much pain in my left knee. I look over, and it's deformed and sticking in, like, sideways.

I had dislocated my knee. They had to come and scoop me up off the street. It was the most pain I can remember having ever, through childbirth or anything, this knee pain was excruciating.

As I'm in the hospital, waiting for the doctor to come see me after the x-rays, after they reduce my knee. I know I'm going to need surgery; I'm waiting for the knee surgeon I had hired, who was previously a spiritual coach. Let me call this man Mr. I-have-no-letters-behind-my-name.

He talked to me. I was having some suffering in my life. At that point, even though I was married and I was happy, I was still feeling a little bit of underlying stress that something was just not quite right.

I hired Mr. I-have-no-letters-behind-my-name, who calls himself the Soul Whisperer, for $8,000 for ten sessions.

I cannot tell you what he did.

But my life just turned around after that.

My business was amazing.

What, why did my life turn around after that? Because Mr. I-have-no-letters-behind-my-name when I was in the hospital called. We had a coaching session, where he said to me, "The reason that this happened to your knee is because you've been inflexible. You have a lot of intuitive abilities, and you're not using them at all. This is why you hurt your knee."

You might call this blaming the victim, but I knew he was right.

Because the previous December, I had a psychic sitting at a table across from me at an entrepreneurial event, tell me, "you have visions, don't you, and you were good."

Then I had a scientific hand analysis with my handprints that showed that I had eight gift markings. Now only ten to fifteen percent of the population has any gift markings in their hands, and I had eight of them.

And she also informed me that five of them were intuitive gifts. If I wasn't using these gifts, then I wasn't on my master path in life.

One knee injury later.

All kinds of undertones of not feeling like I'm doing what I'm supposed to do, running more of a car export business than a medical business.

I decided, and was convinced that I had to come out and talk to people about my ability to read energy, and help them with their health.

It was scary.

Now, yes, of course, I found some mentors, and that's a whole other story. I did find mentors to verify that I could do these energetic readings.

And I realized that I was so accurate.

That I could, by knowing the first name, the last initial, the age, and the sex of someone, read what was going on with them spiritually and emotionally, and link it to what I was seeing that were important factors in real life. Now of course, you have to learn how to talk about these things in non-medical terms. Why? Because doctor colleagues will accuse you of diagnosing and giving medical advice. When you're doing an energetic reading, that's just not allowed.

I tell you this story because, as I got more and more out there in the media, on Facebook, on Instagram, on LinkedIn, other doctors started coming to me behind the scene and saying, "You're good at getting out there, being seen."

"How do you have the courage to do what you do? How do you do those readings?"

My coaching and consulting of practitioners to help them learn how to transform their ticket and do high ticket programs, and raise their own fees, and to read people energetically, and put it in their science-based practice without sounding woo woo became something I started to help people with when practitioners came to me, if they wanted help with their business. It was about getting results. It was about helping them give themselves a raise. But if it was about needing a spiritual awakening, it was about walking them through that, so they can move forward with a different way in life, either in their current practice or in a new direction.

I want you to know, full disclosure, who I am.

You can understand that. I started my ophthalmology practice from patient zero and built it up to double-digit thousands of patients. Almost a million dollars a year working part-time.

A very successful, profitable practice, part-time.

And then I went on to consulting for people's health transformations and consulting for other practices with my colleagues and practitioners, and quickly, within nine months, built up a six-figure business.

The most important piece of information for you to get out of this is that you can also get over your depression, your burnout, your exhaustion, and move forward. In a way, to a new life.

And I'm going to walk you through the steps that I now take my clients through, so that you can decide, should you stay in medicine or should you go.

If you decide that you're going to stay, you can reinvent yourself so that you can find meaning again, and make more money, or you can move on to something else, have your offerings and intellectual property, and feel good again about life, as you spend time with your family and your hobbies and do exactly what you want to do.

Chapter 3

THERE IS A WAY TO MAKE IT ALL BETTER

I know you're at your wit's end right now and you're trying to figure out the best thing to do at this point. You've got all kinds of things going on in your head, but you're also like the deer in the headlights. You're stunned. You're paralyzed. But you know you want to do something. But how do you get where you want to go? And where do you want to go, anyway?

Do you love medicine? Do you hate it? I know that you are just incredibly frustrated and angry on one side, and on the other side, you're feeling miserable because you loved what you did. I loved, loved, loved my patients. The business of medicine? It sucks for doctors...and nurses...and patients. Administrators? Pharmaceutical companies? Health insurers? They are loving it. They are running the show and getting paid. Those of us who care the most are having a lot of hopeless days.

You can get back that feeling of exhilaration about your life and your journey. You are smart and you worked so hard for so many years to get where you are. I want you to be able to celebrate again. I want you to feel happy, and I want you to get paid your value (without being overworked and exhausted). That's why you went for this. That's why you stayed with it and worked those 100-hour weeks for all those years.

If you want to do it differently, medicine or life in general, you are at a crossroads. You must answer a few questions at this point and come up with a plan of action. You must get real and honest with yourself and where you are, and admit if things aren't going as planned. There is a way to get back on track, and here it is. I'm going to take you through the process of getting real and clear, and then developing a plan for your best next move. I'm going to take you by the hand and guide you along the path, to be able to answer the question about what you should do.

After several years of not only coaching health clients in a different way, but coaching practitioner clients, I am like you. I analyze and analyze exactly what I've been able to do, to get results for myself and get where I am today, but also what I've done, to be able to help my clients transform.

And when I'm talking transformation, I'm talking about people getting well, and also people having awakenings and feeling revitalized in their business and practice, or going in a different direction, happily and courageously.

I remember well a couple who were my early clients. They were a married couple in their late fifties. The wife was struggling with being overweight and having multiple food sensitivities, and her husband, an exacting engineer, was struggling with his weight and getting his blood pressure under control, his cholesterol down, and some belly fat he couldn't seem to conquer. When Mr. and Mrs. Cabs (not their real name) charged that $13,900 onto their Discover card (upfront), it put me to the test. Yes, I did get them both major weight loss. Mr. Cabs was able to stop some of his blood pressure meds and Mrs. Cabs was able to understand better what foods to eat and not eat to keep both her food sensitivities and seasonal allergies under control. It felt good to see the major transformation, especially when Mr. and Mrs. Cabs tell me how their primary doctor says to them, "I don't know what you are doing but whatever it is, keep it going."

The revelation is that when people pay, they pay attention. This couple was not simply paying me to guide them. They were investing heavily in themselves in time and money.

It was exhilarating to guide this couple in how to heal themselves using food and botanicals and mindset shifts. Oh boy, the mindset shifts were big as they realized how much power they had.

When people ask me what I do, I want to answer, "I empower people." I would get back the deer in the headlights look if I did answer that way. This is truly empowering work I realize, and I'm in my flow and sweet spot probably for the first time in my life. I'm doing my thing, and people are getting better, and it was oh-so-easy for me to guide them. This coaching thing is Da Bomb!

Let me lay this out for you because I want you to understand that there is hope. Here's how you can get it.

Step One: Plan Your White Space. This is so that you can clear your schedule. You can clear your head.

Step Two: Let's Be Honest. Take a look at the four core areas, the five core areas of your life, to identify where your feelings and strengths are.

Step Three: Find Your Pot of Gold (at the end of the rainbow). This is for you to be able to identify your hidden gifts, talents, and passions outside of your current situation.

Step Four: Put out the Garbage. This is how you see what's holding you back and how to let it go for good.

Step Five: Claim Your Territory. This is when you find an area that's going to be your special area. The skills that you've learned in the past, to transfer them to a new situation or help you move in a new direction.

Step Six: Talk It Out. This is when you learn the few questions and six impactful words that will help you move in the right direction with confidence.

Step Seven: Create Your Passion Protocol. This is when you come up with your secret sauce and learn how to put it into your step-by-step-process that you can offer to people.

Step Eight: Bundle the Bliss. This is where you learn how to give yourself a huge raise by specifically defining your new path and offerings by learning how to name, package, and price your services.

Step Nine: Your C.A.R.E. Solution. This is where you learn the four-step simple flow of life, so that you're able to move forward differently. You will have clarity about what to do and why, who to talk to, how it all translates to money, and then enlisting the exact team of people to help you implement efficiently, so that you stay happy, healthy, and wealthy.

After we go through all the steps, I'm also going to give you a few secrets. I'm going to show you the pitfalls, where people fail, because, yes, there are failures. I've learned to figure out what it is that makes people fail, and I'm going to lay that out for you.

Then, finally, I'm going to tell you how to get the A (and the extra credit to so you have the 4.3 grade point average) because this is what smart doctors do. There's a secret ninja move that can help you do it faster and better.

Chapter 4

HOW TO TAKE BACK YOUR TIME

White Space. Nothingness. That's what I'm talking about. Doing nothing. Planning nothing. Reading nothing. Simply Being, with no plan or agenda except to do nothing at all.

These days, when I ask someone how they are doing, no matter if they're a five-year-old or a retired senior citizen, the answer is the same. "Busy." Doctors are the worst. Not only are most working as part of a practice, but they are also running a committee – a professional one or a community one. They participate on the boards of charities. They're writing a book or a paper. They are presenting at a conference. They're working on another certification. Or better yet, they're running a certification for something else. These are just the male doctors. Female physicians take it to a whole new level, trying to add on Supermom, Superwife, and Superneighbor, all while training for their second Ironman.

I know this because I've been there. Run a practice, home-schooled, taught Sunday school, and trained for marathons and half marathons.

I met my beloved friend, Judy, while training for my first marathon. Of course, I couldn't do just the marathon. A 26.2-mile marathon for no reason wasn't good enough. I had to fundraise and be doing it for a good cause, too. I added on fundraising for the Leukemia and Lymphoma Society. One day, as I was talking with Judy about what I was doing next, she asked me, "Do you ever just BE?" "Huh, Judy? What does 'just BE" mean, exactly?" I ask. She answers "You are always doing. How about you just BE. Do nothing. BE."

She stopped me in my tracks. Simply Being, existing with no particular agenda or not actually planning and doing something, had never even crossed my mind. After all, everyone around me, especially my colleagues, was doing, doing, and doing.

I had been feeling awful. Tired. But I would never admit that to anyone. I had begun to dread everything. That profound question, from a friend that I met running a marathon, sparked the thought of planning my escape so I could, for the first time since probably age four, simply BE.

This is important because it was at this time, when I "escaped," that I first noticed that my head became clear. Suddenly, there was time to think about something other than my practice, my kids, my husband, training for runs, et cetera et cetera and et cetera.

This is the first step. You have to create a White Space on your calendar page.

This is not the same as scheduling a vacation. This does not involve your kids or your spouse. This isn't about going on a mission with Doctors Without Borders. This is time simply for you. it needs to be more than ten days to two weeks.

Think one-month minimum. Optimal is three-months. Why? Because pretty much everything happens in that magical time of about 100 days. Think about how the body resets in about that amount of time, like a hemoglobin A1C. Major change takes about that long when you let it. You don't need a research study to know that what I am telling you is right.

I know that what's probably in your mind at this moment is that you can't do that, and for all the usual reasons (excuses): Money. Familial responsibility. Work responsibility. Whatever excuses you can come up with to resist taking care of you. That is why you must immediately start planning your White Space. You know that no one thinks clearly under stress. Look at your patients. You know what happens to their health because of stress. You tell them they have to do something about it. Now you have to tell yourself the same thing. You have to practice what you preach.

More yoga classes aren't the answer. Going to silent retreats where someone else tells you what to do and what to eat and how to be isn't the answer. You have to be in a space and a vacuum where you can simply allow your system to calm down. You know it will probably take at least two weeks from when you begin this White Space to stop bad-mouthing yourself and start seeing the reasons why this time is productive even though you are doing nothing. Did you hear me? Doing. Nothing.

Dr. Robin was an internist working in a practice for the hospital with three other doctors. She just got tired of having such a high patient load and simply not feeling satisfied in her career. Every day, she was expected to see more patients. The patients were getting sicker and sicker, and in fact, her pay had been stable for the past five years. You know how it goes – more work, more patients, more paperwork, electronic medical records, and all the other things that get heaped on the doctors, and yet the pay stays the same. But what's even worse is that she was spending more and more hours at the office and rarely had any time off. Even when it was scheduled time off, she was coming into the office because she had not finished the work. Dr. Robin decided that she was going to quit. Her next move was something it takes a lot of guts to do, but it's one of the best moves that anyone can make towards getting it figured out. She decided to simplify her life, downsize as much as she could, and go on a vacation for as long as her money would last.

Here's the beauty of her plan. She got a locum tenens physician position and decided to live the life of working vacation to vacation, instead of working where she had four weeks of vacation a year. Four weeks seems like a lot, but is hardly anything when you're working those 100-hour weeks, so think about it. What if you worked for two months and took off one month, and your idea was simply to fund your relaxation and enjoyment. You can do something like this. It's important to think about doing something like this, because you know what happened? Dr. Robin was overweight when she was in her practice and getting larger because she was under so much stress. You know that stress hormones keep the weight on you. You know that cortisol does that to you, plus you're eating junk all the time, and you don't have time to work out. You have no time for self-care.

Dr. Robin saw the writing on the wall. Immediately after she quit, within one year she had lost almost half of her body weight. I had never seen her smile so much. She was a completely different person when she had a smile plastered on her face. I also noticed that those lines that seemed like they were in her forehead all the time weren't even there. Even though she was aging, the lines on her face were going away because that's what happens when you reduce your stress. What would your life look like if you had unlimited amounts of free time and you worked simply to fund your free time? You can do this, and I'm going to talk more about this later on, so you can live a Dr. Robin life. Locum tenens physician might not be the best way for you to do this, but there are definitely other ways that you can do this and even have the type of position where you can work from home, set the hours that you want, and make more money than you did working 100-hour weeks in the office.

How do you do this? Let's address your excuses. These are all the reasons you came up with to keep the status quo. The brain is a lazy organ. It doesn't want to use more glucose and you, even in your burned-out state, will hear your brain telling you all the reasons why you can't do this or why this is stupid or why it won't work for you, or, the typical doctor response, why you can do it in a shorter amount of time. You know, why you can graduate from White Space in two and a half weeks rather than two and a half months You need at least a one-month minimum. You need to plan to do it quickly. Not in a year or two. Within the next six months.

First, go to your family and tell them that you have to do this. Even if you have little kids, you are going to talk to them and say, "I gotta take care of me. You see how I take care of you? I have to take care of me. I'm planning to take some time off from parenting for a bit."

Now here is when you enlist spouses, family, friends, and your community. You speak directly to them and tell them that you are stepping away for a while and that it has to happen within the next six months. If not, you just can't take it anymore, and you'll be a statistic and a story in the paper.

That's right. Be vulnerable to your family and friends. Of course, some will resist. Not your kids, because they love you and understand. Kids are wise and resilient. Stop telling yourself that there will be some harm to them because you took care of you for a time. You must be firm and vulnerable. First, be firm with yourself, so you won't wimp out when, on the verge of your White Space, something happens that you think only you can handle. That's false thinking and your ego fighting you. Somebody's going to get sick. Somebody's going to die. Somebody's going to lose their job. You know what? Those things happen every day, and they get handled. You better stick with the White Space plan.

Second, go to your job and tell them you want paid leave. I don't care if it's a big institution or not. Go ask for paid leave. If they say there is no precedent for that, then great, you are a trailblazer. You have to be willing to draw a line and be courageous. You are at the edge here, and you must let them know that it's either paid leave or goodbye. Now you may need to be more diplomatic. Tell them you are doing a study with a colleague (me) and we are testing the effect on physicians' morale and performance of taking time off when needed and coming back. It's a pilot study. Tell them what you need and that you appreciate their understanding and willingness to help one of their highly esteemed physicians thrive so you can do better for them. Make it a win-win. They have to see what's in it for them. In reality, this is all about you. I'm simply giving you the push to go ask. What is the worst that will happen? Worst case? They'll say no, and then you'll know that they do not care about you. The truth is that good doctors are expensive to find and train. That's why you should plan three to six months out, so they have time to cobble together locum tenens or something. Let them figure it out, but you helping by suggesting how it can work for them will go a long way to getting to "yes" faster.

Be honest about money also. One to three months of time off is not going to topple your finances. If you say, "Yes it will," then it's even more urgent for you to take this break. It will open you up to different ways of doing the money thing, and give you time to figure out how to get things done on a bit less. Everyone else's needs can wait for three months. Don't worry about college tuitions or retirement funds. I want you to dip into those funds for you so that you will be around to enjoy your kids' college graduation and you won't be a broken-down, miserable old person. Make the money thing work. You are smart enough to figure something out. After all, doctors are the penultimate problem solvers. If you don't have it, borrow it from someone or be like the rest of American and get out your credit card. I know I get emails at least once a week offering me lines of credit. If that is what it will take to get you back on track and able to meet your financial obligations like mortgage and car and food, dip in and do it. Invest in yourself. You can pay it back when you get through your exhausted period.

I just addressed the biggest barriers to your White Space. Family. Money. Job. I'm sure you will try to think up something else and tell me how your case is different. Recognize that for what it is – your brain trying to stay with the status quo.

Now, it's six months down the line. You are in your White Space. What do you do? How do you actually BE, exist in the world without doing anything and with no particular agenda? What is going to happen?

You are going to make no plan at all except for how to do as little as possible. Anything that brings up health-harming emotions such as anger, shame, irritation, wimpy and scaredy-cat feelings, or grief, you are going to stop immediately as soon as those feelings come up. You are also going to resist the urge to read anything related to work.

Turn off the TV. Turn off the phone, tablet, and computer for at least eight hours a day. Any emergency that could happen, you are going to assign someone ahead of time to handle. You must have days of nothingness, days you'll spend looking at the walls and seeing what comes up. Be and observe for at least ten days (I'll give you weekends off if you must but preferably not). You are training yourself and others to clearly understand that this time is solely for you to do nothing. Just as much as you must train yourself, all the people around you have likely gotten used to you being the super person they can always go to and bother, and you will always say yes and come to the rescue. You must learn to say "yes" to your own needs, want, and desires and "no" to others. This is the establishing of boundaries that may have never even existed at all in your life, but now are mandatory so you can get yourself on the track you would like to be on. No need to tell anyone exactly what you are doing because the direction is to do nothing. Tell them you have to have time to clear your head. Everyone understands that. What are you doing? Are you clearing your head?

Why? Because this is the real key to the kingdom – for you to overcome exhaustion, fatigue, cynicism, and rest your body, heal your spirit, and rejuvenate your mind,

In this White Space time, you will become reacquainted with you. Get out of the left-brain, logical you and back to the free-flowing creative and playful genius. Fly like a bird. Things will begin to open up for you.

You want to know how much time it takes to open up? There is no study on this. It's different for everyone. Depends on how tightly you are wrapped and how long it takes you to surrender to the joy of Being. You may need to take a stretch and then come back. Your first White Space may need to be repeated. That is okay. Right now, your brain is exhausted, so it is telling you all kinds of crap. Once you emerge from White Space, you'll say, "How did I ever have that kind of thinking?" The thinking that allowed you to descend into a space of spinning your wheels of despair, believing that where you were was the best it would ever get, and that you deserved to be miserable and feel bad, and that working just a little harder, being a little more disciplined, taking on another certification was the way to bliss.

During this time, you will notice that a path for how to proceed in life will start to emerge without you even planning it. It will arise out of the air. The universe will give you answers. Pay close attention to your dreams as your White

Space progresses. Carry a notebook around to write down random thoughts.

Ground yourself. Go outside in bare feet and stand out there. It doesn't matter the time of year. You need to touch the earth as much as possible. Even in the winter. Cold can be invigorating. Go for walks. Without music. Reconnect with all of your senses. What do you see? Notice the beauty in everything. Look at an old person and notice their beauty. Even when their body is betraying them, they have beauty. Notice rocks, trees, flowers, snow, birds, grasshoppers. Notice smells. Pick up dirt and taste it. Yes, it is good to eat dirt. Boosts your immune system. Look. Listen. Touch. Taste. Smell. Feel. Then go in and look again at what's beautiful in your home. Resist any urges to straighten or fix anything the first two weeks of your White Space. No busy-bodying at all allowed. Just BE.

You get an A+ for Being for twelve weeks. An A- for eight weeks. Six weeks equals B, four weeks equals a C, two weeks equals a D, and one week? An F. You think I am being extreme here. First, I'm appealing to the perfectionist side of you. I know you want an A. Let me tell you about one of my favorite master coaches, Dan Sullivan. Dan is a coach to a lot of high-level successful entrepreneurs like Lisa Sasevich, Joe Polish, and Peter Diamandis. Dan talks a lot about the Self Managing Company, and making the goal for entrepreneurs to have as much completely free, untethered time as possible. Dan himself takes about twenty-six weeks a year of completely free time doing exactly what he chooses. You know what this does? It frees his mind to create more innovative ways to help entrepreneurs be successful.

Go for a minimum of C on your first White Space attempt. Trust me on this. If by now you are not trusting me, then close this book and give it to someone else because the rest of what I am going to say isn't going to work without doing step one. This is mandatory. For those of you who stick with it, you will be coming back and telling me stories like Dr. Robin's.

White Space for you is necessary to get to the happiness and more money.

I talked all airy-fairy and business-y technical here, but let me tell you this: White Space is a tantric orgasm. It feels so good and you want it to go on forever. You want to get mad that the pleasure was withheld from you before now, but you feel too good to even have your energy go that way. My client, Dr. Missy, after her first week of White Space was so satisfied, that silly smile on her face as she told me what she had figured out to keep some White Space in her schedule after she restarted working in her practice again. She also let go of the idea that this doing nothing was being lazy. She put out that garbage. I'll help you in a bit put out some of your garbage, and I'm not talking about tidying anything up either.

Chapter 5

TAKE AN INVENTORY SO YOU CAN TAKE CONTROL

Step back and look at where you are. You've come a long way, baby. You have, even if you feel unaccomplished or as if you haven't done enough or aren't where you wanted to be by this point in life.

Here is the secret that no one told you. No one is where they thought they would be. If they say they are, then they're lying. Overachievers always keep raising their bar. The horizon is always moving away and never seems to ever get closer.

Let's get honest and specific about what is going on. Let's get some insight into your case study of one, which is you studying you. This is your self-observation of five core areas of your life, present and future. Your situation is the result of all the decisions and choices you've made up to this point in time.

Health, Career, Finances, Relationships, Spirituality/personal growth – take out your journal (the one you started when you created your White Space) and jot down what comes up for you. Write down the thoughts and the feelings associated with these five core areas.

Most health care practitioners are so busy assessing others and helping others that few have done a deep dive into their own life. You have to commit yourself to at least looking. You are not going to be able to map out the road to success without knowing exactly where you are starting from and having some way to measure your progress.

This is an assessment to do about one time per year. Acknowledge now that this exercise is dynamic. What holds true today and what you need, want, and desire will change over time. As you are on your journey, you will reach goals and set new ones.

Here is what to assess:

Health – where are you today? Where do you want to be in one year? I don't recommend to my clients using long term horizons like two, three, five or ten years at all. From working holistically with my health clients, I have seen major transformations happen within ninety days, so one year is an eon, even if you commit and implement only one little change a month.

When you make your assessment in health, look at what is important, like how you feel and whether you have anything going on that is painful or life-threatening. It's important to not beat yourself up or set up aggressive goals that are based on someone else's standards.

I admire the supermodel Iman. I look at her and at times feel like why I am not six feet tall, slim and gorgeous and glamorous. I could diet to anorexic proportions and over workout trying to look like Iman, and still I could never get there, even when I was fifteen. She is her and I am me. My goal current state? Middle-aged. Fit enough that I can jog at least four miles on any given day, I can do spinning and hit new PRs. I'm no longer a size four. My blood pressure is good. Any aches and pains come from working out harder than I probably should. I take my supplements most days. I drink my tea daily. I consciously think about eating the rainbow of fruits and vegetables. I keep different kinds of green juices in the fridge and have at least one a day. I do like the Rita's gelato and ice cream. I drink alcoholic beverages once a week at no more than two drinks (usually one because my detox pathways are great, and I feel woozy quickly). I keep Pellegrinos on hand so I drink my water. I don't get eight glasses every day. My pee is light though, so I am well hydrated. Coffee I have a two to three times a week.

You see what I am doing here? I'm laying out where I am. I'm not comparing myself to Iman or Gwyneth Paltrow or Julian Michaels or even the other lady doctors in my Peloton Female Physicians Group on Facebook. I admit that I am doing all of this and am peeved that I'm not a size four anymore. Here is the big thing for me though. I feel good. I'm on no pharmaceuticals and have no chronic conditions. I'm grateful for that. Very grateful.

As you lay out where you are, don't compare yourself to me. Say where you are and be grateful that you are strong enough to think about this, and acknowledge how far you've come and that you are still on this side of the ground, not under the dirt, which means there is another chance to take small steps to change.

You probably spend most of your days thinking about health. Maybe even more time worrying about someone else's health instead of your own. The biggest threat to the health of doctors is stress. You know the effects of cortisol, both short and long term. You see it every day in the chronic diseases and acute problems of all of your patients. Stress is at the bottom of every physical illness. I'll let you go to PubMed and look it up yourself, but don't you dare get sidetracked trying to be a contrarian and prove me wrong. Rein in your ego for your own good, Doctor, and go with me.

Which emotional/spiritual issue is at the root of your health problem? Or your illness or your injury? I know something popped up in your mind, even if you immediately wiped it away and said that isn't possible. You know exactly what it is in your life that's "causing" your issues. Now I am using "cause" loosely here. I know the statistical yadda yadda and definition. Drop in with me to those unseen areas that are associated with havoc in your body. Okay, now we know the areas you will have to work on. Pick only one, not a list of every little thing. Let's not get overwhelmed here. Do you know why patients are noncompliant? Because doctors give them so many complicated things to do, they can't succeed, even with the best of intentions. I'm not letting you do that to yourself.

What is the biggest threat to your health? What do you worry about most with your health? What one opportunity is emerging that you can take advantage of to shift your health? Circle the one thing, the one opportunity that you know you can implement. Consider carefully that emotional or spiritual trigger. Right now, simply notice it. Later in the book, we will talk more about transforming this emotional and spiritual trigger from mess to success. (There is a simple process for that. You will be surprised because, as physicians, we are used to everything being complicated and hard.)

Okay on to the boogie man: finances. When you hear the word money, what do you think about? Would you characterize your feelings surrounding money as positive or negative? Be honest. Where are you financially? Where would you like to be in one year? Don't worry about the "how" at this point. Assume that something can change in a positive direction. With that as your assumption, where do you want to be? It may be about paying off debt, or increasing your income or assets and saving for a specific event in a year. What progress would you need to make you feel happy about your finances? Don't mention winning the lottery unless you regularly play, and that is your plan. A lot can happen in a year. Where are you now? What is your major financial goal for a year from today? Be as specific as you can. You know that you have to be able to measure something to be able to come up with a path. We'll get creative with that. (I have achieved an extra six figures in a year, and I've seen friends gain seven figures, but first, you have to believe it in your core and make it your vision before it can happen.)

Career. What are you doing now? Is it exactly what you want to be doing professionally? What exactly would your dream job or career look like? Describe it – money, hours, situation – place everything on the table as possibilities. Write down precisely what you want. Exactly. That is your one-year plan. Off the top of your head, what is the first opportunity that comes to mind that you could take advantage of to achieve that dream career? Write it down. In this area, think about who you might pick up the phone and call that would help move the needle. You have the network – think of one person. Get out their phone number and email, and write it down in your journal.

Relationships. A lot of us have struggled with relationships with our parents, kids, spouse or life partners, and friends. You may even notice that you are feeling alone and isolated. I know how that feels. When my life fell apart, I felt like I knew thousands of people, but no one was there to pick me up. No one was on my team. That's not quite true, but when you are burnt out, depressed, and fatigued, you feel like no one cares. The other side of truth is that you spend too much time at work and on work, and you haven't spent enough time in relationships with a lot of people. You may notice that your circle is tiny, which is why when I said to take White Space, you panicked about who was going to help you.

Let's look at relationship areas. Some relationships may not be applicable. Rate each area from one to ten based on how satisfied you are with your relationship. Use one for unsatisfied and ten for satisfied: Include your mother, father, siblings, children, spouse or life partner(s), and friends. When I crashed and burned, I was below five in all of my relationship areas. There was not one relationship I felt good about. Do you know why?

Because I felt crappy about me. I can't tell you exactly why, except I was always hard on myself. I expected myself to be perfect, and I am still healing from that. I have to thank my friend, Judy, for making me say to myself things like, "I am enough." I also embraced one of Don Miguel Ruiz's Four

Agreements – "Be impeccable with your word." That meant never saying anything negative about myself. Ever. That was life-changing.

You must realize that your relationship with yourself needs to change. This is why I insist that you start with White Space and demand that you ask for and take what you need for You. It is part of your understanding that you deserve it, simply because you are a human being and for no other reason. Pick one of those relationships that score below five and write one thing that you can do to begin to improve it. Remember, it is about doing one small thing at a time, so you can stay in a calm, gentle state with yourself. The energy of the universe will support that.

When I mention spirituality and personal growth in a medical environment that's not full of holistic practitioners, I get funny looks. It's one of those areas that a lot of West-ern-trained doctors don't know what to do with, mostly because we haven't figured out how to study these things with the RCT (Randomized Controlled Trial). I get it in the left, "science-y" side of my brain. But on the other side, at least seventy-five percent of us doctors say we believe in God, Spir-ituality, and the like, and we agree that it's important.

In practice, though, we have become cowards in talking about spirituality and how important it is. I'm not talking religion. I am talking about everyone's connection to a univer-sal source and to each other. I am talking about those quan-tum physics principles that work by a system different than biochemistry and physiology. Many doctors, when they talk to me off the record, admit to mystical experiences in some way. I mean, they know there's something they can't explain, and it's right. Or, they did something that defies medical logic and norms, and it's downright weird, but the patient healed.

This whole area of spirituality is what many patients feels is of utmost concern, even equal to their physical wellbeing. I know that a lot of doctors are burnt out because they feel like they have given up their soul in the way they are forced to practice.

Now is the time to talk about your spiritual state. Whatever it is from nothing to spiritual to a religious system that works (or doesn't work) for you. Where are you? What questions do you have in this area? What would you like to explore over the next year to increase some understanding?

I'll tell you that, when I realized I could read energy (this is my safe way of saying that I am a psychic, okay?), I went on exploring that deeply. Now, in reality, I realized I could do these things long before I said it out loud. In fact, I hid this because I was scared of YOU, my colleagues, ridiculing me. I felt unsafe even though no one knew, and it was in my head. This was a spiritual issue for me that I had to work out. Now, here I am, loving admitting that I am a physician and a psychic. It may be a lot for you to hear right now. Well, too bad if you can't take it. Ignore that I am a psychic. That is MY journey. What is your spiritual state now? Where do you want to be in a year?

I'm going to offer right here for you to get in touch with me if you want to talk about spirituality and personal growth and want a safe place. Remember, I was a Sunday school teacher in a church and hiding that I was psychic, so I have been through my evolution. I'm here to help you through yours.

When Dr. J first started to work with me, she had tried a bunch of other protocols with other doctors to treat her condition. Now, exactly what her condition was wasn't clear to her or any of previous doctors. Dr. J had access to the best and brightest and followed diligently all of their protocols with little to no improvement. After consulting with a well-known mold doctor, it was thought that maybe she was affected by mold even though the testing was equivocal. She was feeling lousy in all kinds of ways. She didn't know where she wanted to go with her career. She had been running a department in a hospital of a major city for several years, and was having some issues in her department with employees getting the work done she had assigned to them. She had an estranged relationship with one of her grown children. She was also the caretaker of one of her adult disabled siblings. She had the nagging feeling that her life wasn't where she wanted it to be. This concern got louder and louder to her as she was moving on in years and starting to think about retirement, but she wasn't quite ready to pack it in yet. As we started to work together, we worked a lot on her spiritual state and what was going on with her relationships with employees, with her children, and with her siblings. We put our heads together to come up with ways for her to handle the challenging employees in a way that felt good for her. Part of this process was for us to do assessments and discuss each of these major areas in life in her life. We worked together for over three months.

She was able to get answers and results in her life because she was willing to step back and look with the microscope at these five areas. It had little to do with the certification she was pursuing. Yes, she was being exposed to mold, but the tests were equivocal. This wasn't the major problem she was having. The major problem was due to ongoing stress – emotional and spiritual stress – due to her familial responsibilities, her past romantic relationships, and her estranged relationship with one of her adult children, as well as her uncertainty about her career, including her challenges with her employees.

As we were working through a physical natural holistic health protocol, we were also working on unlocking what was going on with these other four areas of her life. No, this is not about Psychotherapy – this is about figuring out, in a way, the keys that were important to Dr. J's life. Some of those I was able to see and shed light on, and others had come up for her on her own. Not a big deal about this, as it is not necessarily everything that happened over the ninety days. I was talking to her a year-and-a-half later and found out that she had remarkable clarity in what was happening in each of these areas. She was able to see what was she was going to do with her career, which was to start another section in her department, and have staff colleagues to collaborate with on this.

She was feeling great health-wise, though she was still having some issues with her adult child. But she realized that he would come around when the time was right, and she no longer had high levels of stress and guilt and shame about the state of the relationship. She was able to see that what was happening was that everyone, even her child, was on a spiritual journey that needed to be worked out. She was able to accept what the situation is. This is what happens when you go on these assessments and you start looking at all the five areas of your life. You're able to see where you are and make some plans. Opportunities begin to emerge that you could not see when you first sat down with a blank page, feeling like, "Why am I doing this and what's the purpose of my life?" In the process of healing, it was of utmost importance for Dr. J to be honest with where she was at the point in time when we met, and then take the next step to admit that she needed help. After trying many other practitioners that made logical sense, the best and the brightest, and still not getting a result, she knew that a different process would be necessary to for her to feel better and get focused. The point is that it was necessary for Dr. J to assess and address all areas of her life to get into balance and heal.

Chapter 6

FIND YOUR POT OF GOLD AT THE END OF THE RAINBOW

It doesn't have to be hard. Thinking and analyzing and Googling and agonizing for weeks, months, or even years on end is unnecessary. If fact, taking a lot of time to make any type of shift is generally you getting in your own way of what you want.

Procrastination simply is a sign that you are out of answers. The best way to overcome procrastination is to start in some direction, and only then can you course correct. Your next move right now is to do a trail of what I am telling you. Only then can you decide what is next.

We are going to find your pot of gold. You see, you think it's all about the medicine, and there is nothing else you can do professionally. But there is. Let's look for your gold. Part of this is to get you to realize that some people have multiple life purposes, and they can be wildly divergent. Some things just flow from you. There might have been something in the past that flowed, and there could be something now that is flowing, and you don't even realize it.

I have had "visions" as long as I can remember. They became salient to me about fifteen years ago when I realized that everyone else wasn't seeing stuff like me. I was a practicing eye surgeon – and a clairvoyant. I saw and knew things, like watching a movie. I can envision events in the past, the present, and the future. It is fascinating to me, even now. As these visions came and went, I sometimes felt like I was losing my mind. It was downright bizarre (with a capital B), even to me. I was solidly in the world of medicine, where, if you can't see it, test it, or run a study on it, the phenomenon may as well not even exist. Yet these skills were a large part of what made me a brilliant clinician.

Even back in med school, I could "see" what was going on with a patient. I remember being in internal medicine student rounds with the nail-the students-against the-wall Dr. Dennis Quinlan, and knowing all of the answers so easily. I remember watching his face change when he realized that he could not stump me or mess me up. I remember the smiles on my friends' faces when I gave the answers while all the other students were struggling.

I studied and could ace a test, and I also knew easily and almost instantly what was wrong with someone and what to do, sometimes with no exam or with little or no information.

But I didn't even know I was reading people like this. I couldn't figure out why everyone else thought med school was hard. Or why figuring out what was wrong with people was hard. It was easy for me. I could "see" it and – voilà.

There is something that flows from you. It might be something that you did when you were a kid, and that you were just so good at doing. What did you love to do when you were a kid? Were you great at a sport or music or dance or art or singing? Or perhaps you speak six languages? Go to the mirror and look at yourself. Is there something that you casually mastered that you forgot all about?

Is there something that you love to do now? Like cook? Or organize? You might think it's irrelevant, but how do you know? For example, there is a lady with a large online presence that everybody follows, and a popular show on television. What's her skill? Tidying up. Are you kidding me? We went to med school and worked 100 hours a week, and the world is celebrating cleaning with Zen and Feng Shui. I burst out laughing writing this because, when I see people make a big success by branding some everyday skill like cleaning, I feel like the world is playing a joke on me. But that is my limited thinking, and maybe yours. What I'm getting at is this: is there something that you consider so easy, and maybe even a little bit silly or superfluous, but that you are good at and love?

I do Tae Kwon Do. I started because I was at the studio so much with my kids that I decided to join. Here I am, after going off and on, year in and year out, with a third degree black belt. Part of the appeal of my husband was that he is a Tae Kwon Do master. When we met, I was a first degree and was thinking about starting back. I even got my second degree after an infamous knee injury. Tae Kwon Do helped me get my mojo back and created a goal and balance in my body. It was my focus on passing my second degree testing that made me work so hard in a different way to get my knee healed.

What did you come up with as something that you love? Singing classical opera (I have this dream of being a jazz singer one day)? This is a stream-of-thought exercise, so you can get down on paper those little things that are special about you that you have ignored until now.

Now, tell me, what is so special about your thing? I told you about my psychic thing and my TKD thing. In working with my clients, I use principles from both these parts of me. Both of these skills require incredible focusing of energy. You've seen people who can break a board or a concrete block. That is not physical strength. It is understanding how to move energy and assess energy so that something happens that changes the environment.

Now that you have your special thing, I want you to lay down and close your eyes. We are going to go there. See yourself doing your thing. Make sure you are in your body looking out and doing your thing. What do you see with your eyes? What do you hear? Listen to the sounds carefully. Are you breathing a certain way? What sounds go along with what you're doing in your imaginary enactment? What do you smell? Taste? What does your body feel like? Finally, what emotions are coming forth? Do you feel the joy, the wonder, the exhilaration, the satisfaction of your flow?

I want you to keep on with this feeling for a good fifteen minutes. That feeling of doing something you love. Yes, it could be cleaning with Zen, and it could be your pot of gold or simply something you do for joy. If this activity is something that you haven't done for a long time, how can you get back into it?

Now, if age, time, and money were no factor, what is it that you would be doing? I want you to dream and make it specific, like a 4D experience. It's okay if you want to simply say "travel," just tell me specifically where you would go, what hotel you'd stay in, where would you sit on the plane, what you would see when you go, but here is the thing – that's just a vacation, unless you are suddenly planning to lead trips there or have a retreat there. I want you to imagine life differently and write what it would be like in your journal.

Over the rainbow. At the end of the rainbow. Any way you slice it, anything involving a rainbow is good stuff. If you think about rainbows, they simply appear with ease. There is something that you can do with ease. It could be so easy that sometimes, you feel like a fraud when you do it because it's like, "How easy is this? You mean everyone doesn't know this?"

Well, no. I'm writing this book because a knowledge simply flows and flows from me, so I am sharing it to guide you to a better life. Why? Because part of my life is to see others happy with themselves and in their flow.

A year after she was my client, Katy sent me a note. She had all kinds of strange, rare, and peculiar issues in her body, and she was struggling emotionally with her work and her family. This is a woman who was the responsible high performer in her family and ruled her world. But her world was falling apart because she was having random unexplained symptoms. She had been to the best mold specialist she could find, and to this specialist and that specialist. Still, she found no relief. Someone told her to talk to a medical intuitive. One day, she called my office after seeing one of my advertisements in a restaurant. Somehow, I just knew how to work on her energy. So much so that, even before we met, I sent her a video message, and she said, "I don't know what you did exactly, but I feel better already."

A year later, she was better. Here is her note to me:

"I just wanted you to know that I was thinking how grateful I am to have found you, to have been guided by you, and to be a recipient of your gifts and talents. I'm truly blessed. "

"Wishing you continued love, health, and success."

During our coaching sessions, I had discerned the right questions to ask (through my unique process of doing energetic readings and assessments) on the spiritual front and the appropriate advice to give on the holistic health front so that she was able to have revelations about her career and her relationships with her family and romantic partners, which allowed her to let go of old baggage and move forward. Her nagging health problems were resolved, and she was still going strong over a year after I had last interacted with her.

Isn't this why we became doctors? Because we want to help people like this? And get paid our true value for it? There is a gift or talent you have that can help people, and it is staring you down. It may be something that you take back to the office with you that revitalizes your practice, or it could be something that flows from you and helps people have a whole new life. You see, my pot of gold is also my client's pot of gold. My clients get results because I allow my gifts and talents to flow in an energetic exchange with each of them. It is what I'm meant to give and what they are meant to receive.

When I entered medical school, I could not see that this is what I would be doing. But today, I am using all my skills in this way to help my health clients and my physician clients get to a new place, with the defined systems that came to me through my White Space.

The last part of this phase is for you to decide that you will let go of the limiting belief that this has to be hard and that you need a certificate from somebody to do it. Appoint yourself the authority that you are, in whatever area that you are in. For all the certificates that you have in place, there was that one person who initially claimed the authority and said, "I'm going to make you one, too, so come to my college, med school, law school, program – pay me because I am the authority and I will give you a piece a paper when you finish that says you are an authority, too."

Decide that there is something out there that is absolutely flowing from you and easy for you, that you can bring forth to better your life and the lives of others.

It's time to stop doing it the way others have told you and make your way. This is using the courage muscles that you developed in the White Space with your new flowing creativity and confidence.

Next, we are going to do some housekeeping, so stay with me.

Chapter 7

GET RID OF HEAD TRASH SO YOU CAN FIGURE THINGS OUT

To continue your journey out of confusion and disillusionment, you must let go of some beliefs that are keeping you stuck. I realized that I was brainwashed by the medical education process. Maybe you think brainwashed is a strong word, but think about it. We are taught that if something is not "proven" by a study, then it's not valid. The problem is there are a lot of studies, many we don't even know about, and more coming out every single day. Yet, we have come to believe that we are expected to know every single thing about our specialty or area of expertise.

We cannot know everything; however, we can work on the limiting belief that we have that if something is not published in a journal, it's not valid or not real science. There are so many thoughts and feelings we learn from birth forward about what the world is and what's true. It is our belief system about what is right verses what is wrong that can get in the way of us learning new things and taking a different direction that is better.

In addition to my journey to embrace all of me, including the mystical side, I have also had to study how to practice medicine differently from the way I was trained in medical school. Once I realized I could coach people remotely due to my ability to read energy, I knew I needed to learn more about how to practice this way. I studied homeopathy, functional medicine, and integrative medicine. My goal at first was to help without hurting. Refining my skills and moving energy around to facilitate the healing process was one area of focus. Before I experienced someone else moving my energy, I would have said that this stuff was a farce. But when you experience changes in your body in what seems to be seconds or overnight, and biochemistry and physiology can't explain these "miracles," of course, you think that it is just a coincidence and an anomaly. But people told me how some problem went away after working with me only briefly and energetically. I had to let go of my limiting belief about how the body heals, and that can heal the body.

Step one in putting out the garbage is acknowledging that you have garbage. I call it garbage, because they are someone else's ideas that were programmed into you.

Let's examine. Get out that journal and write down the following list. Next to each word, write down something that you think is absolutely true about that word. Do a free association with this:

- Man
- Woman
- Father
- Mother
- Race
- Ethnicity
- Money
- Lawyer
- Fireman
- Doctor

Next, for each associated word you wrote and assumed to be true, find a case where what you wrote is not true. Are there words where you are resisting finding an example that shows what you thought to be true was false?

Take time doing this exercise. Sometimes it is challenging to find something that contradicts your thoughts.

When you saw the word "doctor," did you think of yourself or someone else? If you thought of someone different, as many people do, perhaps you have never fully embraced your profession, or you are dissociating yourself from it for some reason.

Write everything you can think of that comes up for you surrounding the word "doctor." I want you to revisit the word at least four times over the next twenty-four hours. Keep writing about what is coming up.

The next day, look at the list of associations that you thought were true and those you found to contradict them. Notice what you learned that's new over the last twenty-four hours.

One of the biggest emotions holding us back as physicians is fear. I can tell you first-hand that this was the case for me, and I see it in many of my colleagues. Many of the procedures and protocols of running a practice are meant to keep our fear at bay. This is what we call "CYA medicine." We prescribe according to best practices and standards of care, and we tend not to deviate because we're afraid if we do, there will be a bad outcome, and we'll have to take the fall. What we do every day is serious. We have the lives of people in our hands, and that can be a scary responsibility. There are times when we don't do what our gut tells us because we're fearful. Even though it may be the right answer, if we can't back it up and support it with medical literature or a study, we shy away from it. But is this the way we should live our lives?

Dr. C and I go way back. Sometimes, I'm not quite sure why we stayed friends. Let me tell you, it's been peripheral friendship because our lives have been busy, and only intersect like once every few years because life is just too busy for Dr. C to make time for an old friend who must not be a friend because it isn't all that important to make time for that superfluous thing called friendship. Dr. C has the Physician Perfectionist Personality Disorder (it's like a virus. It's almost impossible to go through medical training without catching it, and no one is researching the cure). I always admired that he could stay so focused and on the path when I've felt like I was falling off the path. Life for doctors like him in a procedure-based profession with a steady flow of sick patients who always need you means Dr. C is doing quite well with all the accoutrements of life. Nice wife. Nice house. Late-model super expensive cars. Vacations in exotic places. He's getting paid well. Dr. C reflected to me on one of our speed say-hi-because-I'm-too-busy-to-slow-down sessions that it is important to have friends that go way back and that keep in contact with him even when he isn't reciprocating so well. Here is what worries me. Dr C recently has developed a hardcore serious "appreciation" for wine collecting (and drinking). The red flag is at the top of the pole and full mast, because, as far back as I go back with Dr C, he was one of the few people who didn't drink. I observed, when we were going out for dinner on one of the few times he wasn't too swamped with work, he had ordered several drinks (not green juice either) during the meal that spanned less than two hours. He confessed that he was just counting the years until he could just get out and retire. Eight more years. That's all he had to get through. Then, finally, maybe he could scale back.

Change is scary, and so rather than make any change, it was just easier for him to pick up a bit more of the bottle (no dysfunction because it still only at night right?). In his state of lasting until he could stop, it wasn't an option to admit that things are not going all that well on the inside even if everything looked stellar from the outside. To admit to himself, his wife, his family, his colleagues, that he wasn't happy in his life and not happy in his career? This is a heart attack waiting to happen. Even though he had all the accoutrements of success, instead of saying, "I'm going to get out of this – I'm going to do something different," he simply picked up the bottle. This is not to condemn Dr. C. I'm scared for him because I don't know if he is going to make it through those eight years with sound body and mind. Substance abuse is an issue that good doctors pick up in their career. To relax. To calm. To numb

Another friend, an OBGYN I've known for several years, called me two years ago and told me that he had lost his license from drinking. He was also in the midst of his second divorce. He was having major health problems. His career, his personal life, and his body were falling apart.

As I tell these stories, I'm sure somebody comes to mind. You may be seeing yourself on their same trail. Take steps to get over the fear and get help. An important reason I'm writing this book is to let you know that I'm here to help. There are other people, including other doctors who have made it their life's work out to help you and protect you and your identity.

We want you to be able to function and be happy again. I don't want you to become an alcoholic or a drug addict. I don't want you to lose another marriage. I don't want you to lose your license and your career. I don't want you to end up having a mental breakdown or killing yourself. I'm in the Club of Doctorhood with you, and I want all of the members of the club to soar together.

The biggest piece of trash you're going to need to take out of your head and put out is your fear.

Let's talk about putting some of our fear out with the garbage. Can we put out all our fears? Can we put out the fear of going against what our mother would have said or what our father would have said? Can we put out the fear of what our spouse might say or do? Can we put out the fear of losing our license? Can we put out the fear of what our colleagues will say? Can we put out the fear of shame? Can we put out the fear of losing our money, our house, our kids, our spouse? What fears can you put out in the trash? Is there a way that you can move forward in some areas of your life by putting the fear behind you? What's the worst-case scenario? And remind yourself of what fear is. Fear is us projecting a negative outcome into the future. You may think, "I'm being careful," or, "I'm just being realistic," or, "I'm just working to foresee problems and ward them off." Truth is, none of us know the future, and even when we truly believe we are in control and that we have planned for everything, something we never even thought possible happens.

Mary lost her twelve-year-old son in a car crash. I had seen Mary two weeks before this at an event. We became friends from spending time in a small group called Mastermind. We were both working on our businesses and laying out our successes and our struggles. At the time we met, we were both writing our books.

Mary had a Facebook account, and I loved seeing her there. I enjoyed watching her live her life, with her son and daughter, and work her business. Mary was hard on herself. She had been through some health issues and, as a result, came up with a company that helped people with health issues. One day, as I scrolled on Facebook, I saw the announcement of her son's passing. There was a date and time and place. That's how I found out her son had died. It was one of those moments when the news is so bad, you lose your breath.

Over the next ten months, I watched Mary work through her grief. She decided to live it out publicly on Facebook. She talked about her feelings, showed her daughter, reacted to the comments that people would make about how she should (and shouldn't) act or feel surrounding her son's death. It's interesting how those brief snippets of her life on Facebook brought out so much emotion in me. There were days when I would sit and cry. I feel joyful watching as Mary is discovering her new normal.

One day, Mary talked about fear in a profound way. She was rollerblading, and one of her friends told her she should be wearing a helmet. Mary told us how she'd lived her whole life not wearing a helmet for skiing, riding bikes, and other sports. But, because suddenly helmets are mandated, her whole life and her kids' lives, even her son who died, had to change because people said you must wear a helmet, even though that's not what killed him. Mary never wore a helmet, she's alive, and she decided she was not going to do something for someone else's fear.

She said, "I'm not going to change the way I live because you're uncomfortable, and I'm going to do exactly what I want to do." Thank you, Mary, for not living in fear and for realizing that you never know what's going to be. There's no need to live in fear. You don't know what's going to happen. Can you put out some of the fear? Can you put it out and do what you feel is right for your patients, even if it doesn't follow best practices, standard procedure, or protocol, but because the universe or whatever you tap into tells you that this is right, and it's going to work, and help the person We need to start doing the right thing for ourselves and for others and put fear out in the garbage.

The other piece that I want you to understand before you go on to the next step is brain gymnastics. Gymnastics of the brain are so important because they help you become more flexible in your thinking. It opens you up to possibilities. One thing that happens in medical training is that we're led down an absolute path, and we become inflexible. There are so many different ways that someone can get better and heal. Many times, we are unwilling to embrace other ways to help people heal; we need to understand that anything that heals the patient is medicine.

My husband's from West Africa, and every once in a while, he sends me videos of interesting events taking place in Africa. One day, he sent me a video of a tribesman in the bush doing brain surgery. This was so fascinating to me, to watch open brain surgery in a non-sterile environment with an awake patient. Suddenly, the brain surgeon and his assistants took a break, in the middle of the operation, to smoke and drink. Seeing the patient with her brain open while they took a break was beyond my comprehension.

I noticed that the narrator was calling this brain surgeon, a "witch doctor." The witch doctor we saw in the video – this brain surgeon – had operated on other people. He is a Bushman who happened to have a high level of skill and the ability to help people. He didn't have a certification; he didn't have a sterile operating room; he wasn't reading studies to decide how to do his procedure. He had obviously been taught by someone who had passed these skills down to him. He was skilled at performing this procedure that helped people heal. We need to understand there are many ways to get there, and we need to be flexible in our thinking. Flexible thinking is something that needs to be practiced. We must put ourselves in different places in different situations so that we see more possibilities and become more flexible. The old saying is true – there are many ways to skin a cat.

Make it a routine to examine if you're piling up brain trash and need to put it out. To get unstuck, you're going to have to put out the trash and do some brain gymnastics, so that you'll have flexible thinking. Yes, continue to question everything, but also look for alternative answers, and realize those answers may not be in PubMed. They may be in a video where you watch a shaman doing something that you thought wasn't possible, and you may even realize that it is real, but a completely different reality than you ever knew existed. Everyone creates their own reality, and everyone's reality is different.

Chapter 8

CLAIM YOUR TERRITORY

You're going to enjoy this next phase of the journey. You're going to get to do something outward that later, you will be able to see.

I want you to claim your territory. You are going to put up a flag.

Let's step back and see what you didn't put out with the garbage. Let's dust that asset off and examine what it is.

Is there something you are seriously good at that differentiates you, that is unique and distinct about you? Something that is wrapped up in the fabric of you that you were just made for?

For me, it is guiding people to clarity and helping people to see better. I had a career as an ophthalmologist. I embraced my clairvoyant side. My tagline on my cards and letterhead, when I had my eye care practice, was "Good vision improves your outlook." In my practice, I would help people improve their vision by prescribing glasses, using lasers to halt blinding eye diseases, removing cataracts, and performing glaucoma surgeries. That time was all about caring for people's sight physically.

As I transitioned into holistic practice, I began to help people gain better insight into how to leave disease behind and create health. I lead clients through health transitions, career transitions, and spiritual transformation, guiding them to have good vision, so they have clarity and focus in their life.

There's something that you're good at, and I want you to claim it. It could be something that you have done in your practice but could also be something that you've done in your life. There's a common thread or a theme that runs through my life, and it's all about vision. It's about seeing clearly. That part of my life was focused on getting people clearer physical vision. I would prescribe glasses. I would treat eye diseases. I would even use lasers and surgery to help people either stop visual loss or regain vision that they lost.

Imagine what it's like to be able to take out a cataract for someone who then goes from not being able to read an eye chart to reading from the bottom row. That was the first portion of my life, but I've transitioned to a new stage. This stage is still about good vision and helping people improve their outlook. But these days, I'm doing things like writing this book to do that. I work with clients to help them have clarity by seeing what the best next step is in their life and implementing it with confidence and clarity. I also help people see energetically. A lot of people consider this strange; however, it has helped me to help my clients work out situations that are strange, rare, peculiar, or difficult.

Is there something in your life that is a common thread? Is there something that's unusual about you, like my "Clairvoyant Eye Doctor?" I want you to glean whatever it is. The weirder, the better. Look at your specialty. Look at what you've done in your career or in your family, or as a child. I want you to stake a claim, put a flag in it, and be whoever that is. This is important because it's part of your story. Remember, everybody loves a good story. People buy from people, and I want you to get to the point where you're able to go out there with confidence. People are going to buy you and what you have to offer.

There's something unique about you, and you may not even see it. Other people may be telling you about it. Here's a real-life example. When, I was the face of American Car Exporters, what began to happen was that people I dealt with all over the world would Google my name and discover I was a doctor. They would text me asking for medical help, and I started to realize my deep skill as an intuitive and a clairvoyant. From just looking at a text message, I could "see" what was wrong with someone. At first, it was startling. But it was also fascinating. How did I verify I knew what was wrong? I began to ask questions of the person to verify that I had gotten the problem right. Simply from their text message asking for help, I knew what was wrong with the person. This is a skill called "claircognizance."

You may have claircognizance without realizing it. Maybe it was something that you felt, where you had an intuitive knowledge, but there was no logical reason you should know this. American Car Exporters led me to embrace my intuitive abilities. These people from all over the world asked for my help as a doctor, and I knew I could help them. It jumpstarted my career as a psychic. I added holistic practice skills when, in my coaching of people, I needed to create a plan for what I was going to do for them. I needed plans they could implement wherever they were in the world, and this is how I've gotten more and more training in holistic fields, such as homeopathy, functional medicine, and integrative medicine.

People know me as a licensed physician and practicing psychic that helps people with problems that are strange, rare, and peculiar. I ended up coaching practitioners, too, because so many people came to me asking how I do what I do. "Can you show me that? How do you have the courage and the boldness to go out there?" Well, guess what? I'm a natural teacher, and I embraced my journey to help all kinds of people see better, whether the people are clients with a health crisis or practitioner with a life or a practice crisis. My goal is to have more people and more practitioners who are like me. When I go someplace, and people say to me, "Why aren't there more doctors like you?" What I can say now is that I'm working on it. I'm not saying that you have to become a psychic, but there is something you're good at, that you can use to help a lot of people.

There was a back surgeon, Dr. John Sarno, who realized that, when he operated on people who came to his office with back pain, the surgeries always seemed to go well. But this had nothing to do with his skill as a surgeon. After his surgeries, some people continued to have pain, and some didn't. What he realized was that the people who still had pain, and continued to have pain, were also having emotional issues. If he helped people work through those emotional issues first, he found they often did not need to have back surgery.

Now, a lot of his colleagues thought that he was utterly crazy, They labeled his ideas as "unscientific and simplistic." His response was, "I don't have to prove anything to you, my medical colleagues. My proof is the patients who are getting well and healing." He's right. There is an entire website devoted to thanking him from the people who have read his book and worked with him.

Two take-aways from me and Dr. Sarno:

1. Doing the inner work, the spiritual and emotional work, can heal your body and your life.

2. Forget what your colleagues say, and do the right thing to help people, even if it seems bizarre by others' standards

What I would like you to embrace is the side of you that has to go out and claim your territory in another area, one that is peripherally related to what you do. A territory where you can be known. Here's where you get to do something fun. First, I'm going to walk you into claiming your territory. Your assignment is to go out and have a photoshoot.

You're asking, "Why are you telling me to go out and have a photoshoot?" Because I need you to embrace the new you, and you're going to do this with a photoshoot. You're saying, "Photoshoot. This is completely out of my comfort zone, out of my wheelhouse." Good. This whole journey is about getting you out of your comfort zone so that you can be preeminent in your next phase of life. People will buy you, your employer's going to buy you, and they'll pay you more money. Or you're going to strike out on your own, ask for what your true value is, and have the life that you want. You're at the point right now where you're going to decide who you want to be, where you want to be, if you want to stay in medicine, or if you want to go.

You know enough now that, whether you want to stay or go, either you're reading what I'm saying and want to get back to what you're doing, or you're reading what I'm saying and are excited enough to say, "I'm ready to jump." I don't want to help you jump. When I jumped, there was no one and nothing at the bottom to catch me. I want to be your net and transition you even if you're going to stay. Whether you decide, "This isn't for me, I'm ready to go back, I love medicine a whole lot," or you decide, "I'm going on this journey, I love medicine."

You are going to go and have this photoshoot. Present the different face of you because even after reading only a portion of the book, there is already a different face of you, a different part of you. Here's what you need to do. There are lots of apps you can go out and look at, or you can ask around. I don't want you just to get a headshot. I want you to have a complete photoshoot, even if you're a man. That means hair and makeup and outfit changes. I want you to have fun with it. I want you to go outside, I want you to go inside, or you may want to do something like fly to New York or fly to LA. Make this a fun production, hire a stylist to help you put together some outfits. There are stylists out there that can help you on a budget, or take you to 5th Avenue, and put you together that way. Wherever it is, whatever your taste, you can put this together. I want you to hire someone to do your hair, and someone to do your makeup (even if you're a man) because this is what's going to make you look back later at wonderful pictures. Know this; it's going to be a fun half-day or full-day for you. I want you to think of it as fun because you're putting the new you forward. Think of yourself as if you're the superhero in the cape whenever you're doing a posing. Have fun with it. It's you and your team, and they're there to take care of you and make sure the best you comes forward in the photos. When you look at yourself, you look back and say, "Oh, my God, I look wonderful."

Now, don't tell me you'll do it when you lose five more pounds, or you'll do it when this happens or that happens. No, I want you to plan for it now. Schedule it within the next thirty days. Put together the team. Get black and whites, get colors, because you're going to come back with seven or eight hundred pictures. The next time someone asks you for a picture, you're going to have an array of different pictures of yourself that you can present to convey what you want to convey at that time. Don't think about it.

You look at a website – let's say a hospital website – and what do you see? Boring, boring, boring pictures. You believe that, when they look boring, it makes you look trustworthy, but it's all just so cookie-cutter. You want to put your personality in it. I'm not saying don't use a suit, or don't wear a jacket or tie. I want your pictures to show you in different colors, different styles, dressed up, dressed down, casual, jeans, or whatever. Have a variety of different looks and styles.

Know what else you are going to do with these pictures? You're going to buy a URL, a web address for you and your name. For instance, you know me as DrVeronica.com. Find your web address, and make sure it's a.com. You can find it somewhere, even if you have a common name. Put a "doctor" in front of it or put your credentials behind it to make it unique. You're going to buy the URL so that you can put your pictures up on a website.

I don't want you to do any other website building at this time, but I want you to claim the URL for your brand. For the rest of your life, it's going to be your creation, so whether you go back and work in your practice or your hospital, or you go forward into some type of new business, whether it be in health-related field or something else, you have your unique name and your brand.

You are claiming your territory now. You may say, "I've got to think about it, I've got to ask people…" No, this is not what you're going to do, you're not going to think, you're not going to ask, you're going to go with your first thing up. Here's what I'd like to do – don't get scared – this is the point where people get scared because they're like, what if I claim the wrong thing?

Don't worry, it's not permanent. I want you to try it on for size for at least six months. What does it feel like to be whatever you are? What does it feel like for you to be Dr. Mariah, the Psoriasis Solver? What does it feel like to be Dr. Regina, the Statin Buster? You can be playful with this because people are going to remember it about you. What if people are coming to you because you are the Stain Buster or the Psoriasis Solver? Let's talk about that a little bit more deeply.

I know what is streaming through you head right about now; "But I can do more than just treat psoriasis well. I can do so many other things." Here is where you need to trust the process of claiming your territory. As the Psoriasis Solver, someone is going to come to you and say, "I see that you're excellent at solving psoriasis. I have eczema, can you help me with eczema?" Why, yes, you can. This is how people come to you. You talk specifically to one person, then other people will say, "Can you help me with this?" If it is something else in your skill-set, you're going to be using words that are still going to be hitting on that other person. I know that you know what you're doing. You're going to have people with conditions other than psoriasis come forth to you.

My core genius has become helping practitioners with mystical lives and experience to incorporate that into their practice. Why? I have doctors come to me behind the scenes (on Facebook Messenger and at conferences) and say "I see you do these psychic readings. Can you teach me how to do those readings? How do you talk about it with your patients? How do you market it, charge for it, and make it into a part of your business?"

I'll talk more about making it into a business later. That's definitely coming down the line because I have to spell it out enough so you can see yourself doing it and capture your "thing" into a business model that allows you to put yourself out there and get compensated well for the value that you will be providing to people, finally.

Here is another way to come up with your area of expertise and specialty where you can help people: examine illnesses and injuries.

I've been through physician burnout, so now I can talk about burnout to all kinds of people. I'm the same me, but it's about burnout, which is stress on steroids. Have you been through depression? I have. I can talk to people, and help people through a depression crisis alongside of others on their team. You're saying, "But I'm not a psychologist or psychiatrist." Look at the self-proclaimed experts on just about anything that have little or no formal education in a particular area, who are educating people on strategies to get a transformation. Training and credentials don't necessarily translate to results for clients. There are some health coaches I know making $250,000 a year, more than many doctors, because they've been through their own health crisis, and now coach others better than many doctors. Doctors who simply don't know how to coach, or doctors who think coaching is not a modality that will help their patients. There are whole industries out there that serve people to get results in their health. A lot of doctors are mad (and jealous) that lay people are now getting paid to solve health issues that are not being solved by the conventional healthcare system. The clients that pay these health coaches haven't gotten answers or relief from their own doctors.

You are a doctor with real educational background and training that you can parlay into a different area and in a different way, as long as you don't hold yourself back. There are some logistics involved in making this come together, but first, you have to dream it up and give yourself permission to be creative in the name of helping people. I've been through depression, I've been through burnout, so guess what I've come up with? A system that works, and helps people, because I examined the steps I went through to resolve my crisis, and can use that experience to guide others out of crisis. I wrote it down and claimed the territory of burnout recovery specialist. I've even been on ABC TV as a burnout recovery specialist. Examine illnesses and injuries, and write down how you can help someone get out of a pickle by guiding them through your process.

Examine your spiritual life. Is there something in that area where you can help people and guide them through? In 1998, The Accreditation Council for Continuing Medical Education (ACCME) mandated that doctors learn how to take a spiritual history. How many doctors are actual taking a spiritual history or even talking about it with their patients? This is more than asking what religion someone follows. Patients say their biggest concern is in spiritual and emotional issues when they are interacting in the healthcare system, and this is not only at the end of their life or on their deathbed. Many are interested in understanding the messages and meanings of their illnesses and injuries.

There's probably an area, because you've seen it a lot from the emotional and spiritual state of either your patients or yourself or your family, that you are uniquely set aside to help people through. No, I'm not saying you should administer psychotherapy. I'm saying you can come up with a system to coach people through a type of crisis that will help them get results in their life, without giving medicine, without doing psychotherapy, and without doing a medical diagnosis, and this is a service that can be separate from whatever practice you're in right now. This is something that, if you're in a hospital setting or you're in a large practice setting, you can add as a service to your practice that will help to distinguish your particular practice. But I want to think about this with you first, and brand you with it. You're going to do some test pilots with it, you're going to reach out to some people and say, "Hey, I'm testing this out and I want to talk to you about it," and you're going to work out your system with others and find out whether it's good or not.

As I was working out all of my systems, I've always reached out to people, saying I'm working on this, asking questions, and interviewing people. I find out what their struggles are and tell them what I've come up with. That way, I get verification of feedback that what I'm doing is something that's good and useful, and that's what you're going to do when you're claiming your territory.

Write it down your territory because you are going to embrace it for at least six months, knowing that it could be changed. You may not be able to do this right now. You may have to sleep on this for a few days. Claim your territory in ten words or less, and describe exactly how you can help people uniquely.

Here is a bit more guidance in this area; think about a patient you absolutely love working with. Think of their name, and who they are – an actual patient that you love because there's just something about their personality and the way they are that gels with you. You enjoy seeing them; you were able to help them through their problem, so that you were happy and they were happy. Find that patient in your memory and write down their name. What is it that they had that you helped them through? That may be the exact area that is your genius. I want you to get granular about that person's emotional and spiritual state and their life circumstance. Not simply their physical issues. I don't want you to say, "Well, they had a heart arrhythmia and I helped him through that." There was something else different and special about that person that I want you to grab on to, because there's going to be something about that situation that you are going to use.

Next, go to the other side. Who was your nightmare patient? That person that came in and you didn't like them. They didn't like you. They were complicated and the situation went down the tubes and sideways in a bad way. Things were horrible. What is the name of that person? What happened? This is important to know, because there's certain people and patients that you just don't want to work with. You have to identify those characteristics so that when you're claiming your territory, you know who you want to work with and who you don't want to work with. Look at those qualities, the condition or the personality, or whatever it was in that nightmare situation, and write the opposite of that in the quality. That way, you'll know exactly what you're creating, who you want to work with, and who is in your wheelhouse. At this point, when you have claimed your territory, if somebody walks in that is like the nightmare, you're not going to work with them. You're going to pass them off to a colleague.

Pay attention, because this is important and a concept that doctors are rarely taught. Every patient deserves to be someone's "A" patient. If they're an "F" patient for you, you must pass them on to someone else. You have a moral and ethical obligation to pass them to another practitioner where they can be an "A" patient or client. Stop working with "F"s. Work only with "A"s, maybe a few "B"s.

I reiterate, nothing is permanent. You can change whatever you first come up with. In fact, you will change, but only after you have had enough time to test the bounds of your new territory. That means you have to go into the territory. It doesn't get fleshed out in your head. It gets fleshed out while you are in the territory. Test it out for a minimum of six months (realizing this is a short trial). See and feel what it's like to walk around in your new territory. Put up your flag, because it's your promised land now.

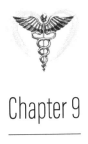

Chapter 9

TALK IT OUT

HOW TO GET EVERYONE ON BOARD WITH YOUR PLAN

Words are powerful. You need to use them carefully. You need to understand them in a different way. One way is to ask good and specific questions. The second is to observe the emotions that are coming out of the answers, using the six main emotional words to describe them.

In talking it out, I want to give you a tool to stop over-analyzing. I don't want you to go off to Doctor Google and do research. I want you to ask a question and then answer the question. Let me show you a technique which is called inspired writing. I'm not sure where I first heard about inspired writing, but this works. You're going to ask a question, write it down, and, in order to tap into your gut and your intuition, you're going to answer the question by writing with your left hand. Your right hand is for logic; your left hand is for intuition. I want you to use this technique so you begin to reacquaint yourself with your intuition. Then, you can tap into it anytime, even when you're not writing. Notice the feelings that are coming up as you're writing answers with your left hand.

Here's the first question I would like to ask you: are you open to doing things in a different way? This is a question you can use with yourself and with any patients or clients you have in the future. After learning these techniques and reading, you're going to want to use these tools to help your patients and clients transform. Why this question? This is the Einstein thing. People keep doing the same thing over and over and expecting a different result. If they're not open to doing things in a different way, they're going to continue to get the same result. Some people want to continue to do things in the same way. The only way you will know this is if you directly ask a question and they answer it – yes or no.

Are you open to doing things in a different way? There's no 'maybe' in this. 'Maybe' is not an acceptable answer. Answering "maybe" is hedging bets. 'Maybe' means, "Tell me what it is, and if I like it, maybe I'll say yes, maybe I'll say no. If I don't like it, I'll say no, but I'm not in a place where I want to move forward so much that the answer is yes. If your client doesn't answer yes immediately, they're not ready to move on. If you don't answer yes immediately, you're not there. That's okay. When you answer yes to this question, you open yourself up to possibility. Or if you are the one asking the question, this is a time when you find out if a person is willing to partner with you rather than you being an authority figure. To get results, a partnership has more impact than you acting as an authority figure and having people do exactly what you tell them to do. This is how collaboration opens up.

Let's talk about emotions. We're going to make this simple. There are six emotions I want you to know intimately for yourself and anyone you work with in the future. I want you to begin to train yourself, when you walk into a room with someone, to assess which of these six emotions they are in without asking a question. You can do this because you're already doing it, but this is where you make it a conscious process.

There are three health-harming emotions and three health-promoting emotions. Health-harming emotions are fear, anger, and sadness. Health-promoting emotions are gratitude, love, and joy. As you continue to go through this book and reread parts, I want you to notice which of these emotions is coming up for you. In the beginning, you came to this book with a lot of confusion. You came to this book with a life-altering question – is it time for you to quit medicine? At that point, you may have been experiencing all three of those big health-harming emotions. If you are suffering from burnout, one or all of these health-harming emotions have overtaken your being. You're fearful of what's coming up next, and whether you can handle it or not. You're angry that you feel unappreciated and unsupported. You're sad because you love what you do so much, and you feel isolated. There may be another combination of reasons behind the different emotions. You can mix it up, but when you came and asked your two questions, you wanted answers to feel better and to decrease your fear, anger, or sadness.

I know when I left medicine, I was angry. I had made a lot of sacrifices. I remember going through the fourth year of medical school, pregnant and hiding my pregnancy, so I would get the residency that I wanted. Residency programs are not prone to select pregnant women to be in their programs. Having a child immediately before or during medical training means scheduling headaches for the programs and more work for everyone else in the program when you are out to have your child or take care of your child in the case of an illness.

I went through my internship with an infant and while pregnant with my second child. I went into pre-term labor nine weeks before the due date. I had put the life of my child in jeopardy because of my dedication to helping people. When I got out, and I was in practice, not enough people said thank you. Not enough people wanted to pay their bill. I missed time with my family. I missed birthday parties. I missed events. I missed all of my twenties and some of my thirties, and I was angry that I made so many sacrifices. I felt I wasn't being appreciated or valued in the healthcare system. Fear was a big part of what I was feeling. I didn't know where to turn. I was having these strong emotions, feeling like I just couldn't take it anymore, and I just wanted to scream, holler, kick, and cry in the middle of my office. I didn't know who to talk to or how to work it out, and I felt there wasn't a soul in the world who understood what I was going through.

The healthcare system is a dog-eat-dog world, competitive. You cannot show your weaknesses or your wounds to your competitors because you'll become the prey of the predators, and nothing excites predators more. Grief and sadness were a big part of my emotions. It wasn't what I thought it was going to be at all. I felt empty almost from the beginning because the system is soulless. Since I was four years old, I wanted to be a doctor, and I achieved that. I did the best I could possibly do, and every day, in my office, in the operating room, in whatever situation I was in, I always gave the best. Now, I was going to have to let it go because it was eating me from the inside out.

As you go through this profound decision about whether you're going to stay or go, and you begin to see how you're going to do that, I want you to examine some of the questions surrounding fear, anger, and sadness. What are your objections and fears about leaving medicine? What is holding you back from leaving medicine? What will your life look like if you don't leave medicine? What will your life look like if you do?

As you assess any situation, and you help your patients and clients assess situations, these are questions you can ask.

The three words, when you boil it down to your negative emotions, are fear, anger, and sadness. Which one is it, and what's behind it?

There are three health-promoting emotions. They are gratitude, love, and joy. Notice that anyone you meet who is well in body, mind, and spirit is usually in a state of gratitude, love, or joy. I know you're saying, "But which came first – the chicken or the egg?" When you met ill patients, they were fearful, angry, and sad. You even look at yourself with fear, anger, or sadness. It doesn't matter which came first – the emotion or the situation. The question is, where are you at least fifty-one percent of the time? When you are emotionally fatigued and burned out, you're in the fifty-one percent of fear, anger, and sadness. When you're in top form, you're greater than fifty-one percent of gratitude, love, and joy. In order to walk strongly and confidently, gratitude, love, and joy must rule the day.

How do you turn a negative into a positive? How do you transform your feelings and your thinking? First, are you willing to do things differently? Are you willing to accept the responsibility that you create your emotions? Are you willing to realize that you can choose how you feel about a particular situation? An event or situation is just that – it's neither good nor bad – it just is. It's the emotion and reaction you choose that makes it either good or bad and takes it out of neutral. When you label it with something that will create fear, anger, or sadness, it takes on that negative spin. When you label it with something more positive, it takes on the energy of gratitude, love, and joy. I want to remind you, if you think what I'm saying is silly, go back to studying the cortisol system. You'll realize that emotional stress is equal to having one or more of the feelings of fear, anger, or sadness about a situation and/or event. Holding on to these emotions, long-term means that it's lodged somewhere in your body. Think about that. You call it a feeling because when you have an emotion, your body feels it and you have a physical reaction. I'm breaking this down simply for you because it's a reminder. I know you're a smart person, and you are ready to know these things, but it's worth pointing it out to bring it to the top of your awareness.

This is what you're going to do. To transform your fear or anger or sadness into the positive of gratitude, love, and joy, you're going to recognize that, whatever it is, the event itself is neutral. Even if it's something that looks like it's going to instill fear, anger, or sadness, you can look at that event and say, "I have gratitude for it, because of the good that can come out of it." When you were in fear, anger, and sadness, something led you to read this book as a way to get relief from those emotions. Has some good come out of that so far? Maybe you've gotten this far along this journey, and you're already happy because you're starting to become clearer about what's going on. Maybe you've made a major shift. By this point in the journey, many clients have already had some fabulous things happen in their life, before they've even finished. I one-upped you to reach out to me about the fabulous things that have happened in your life already before you even get to the end of this nine-step process. I do that because I know they have. Time and time again, when people decide that they are ready to do things differently, they open themselves up, and the universe simply provides. I can't explain how or why.

I would go into a discussion about the laws of attraction, but I don't want to do that right here. I already know that I don't have to explain why. It's like, if I throw a book off a building, gravity's going to happen. The book is going to hit the ground. I don't need to explain the laws of gravity to you. It just is going to happen, whether you understand why or not. When you open yourself up to doing things differently, the universe meets you. That doesn't mean all obstacles go away and everything's a straight line. But once you decided you wanted to experience gratitude, love, and joy, you wanted to be out of pain, you wanted to be out of fear, anger, and sadness (because that's what pain is – pain is an emotion of fear, anger, sadness going on in your body), you decided to pick up this book.

The first thing you need to do is name the main emotion associated with whatever you were experiencing. Think of an event going on in your life, or an obstacle that you think is particularly difficult to deal with. Which emotion is predominant? Is it fear? Is it anger? Is it sadness? You've done the first part of the process. You identified a stressful event or situation, and you've identified the emotion attached to it.

The next step is to write down five ways this situation or event that you're dealing with is good. Write down those ways in which something positive came out of the situation that you see as stressful. Go ahead, force yourself to do this. This is another time where you can use your left-hand inspired writing to connect with your right brain. Writing with you right hand will access your logical left brain; however, writing with your left hand will access your right intuitive brain. You're not necessarily going to be able to come up with the answer with logic. I want you to get out of that and get into your right brain, your intuitive brain that has untapped areas of creativity and brilliance, to grasp why you are on the journey. Every situation that happens to you is meant to teach you lessons. If you don't learn the lessons, the situations that come up become more and more and more challenging and painful. When you learn the lesson and figure it out, pain or fear, anger, and sadness can be easily flipped over to gratitude, love, and joy.

I'm sure you've heard patients say that their illness was the best thing to happen to them. Have you ever heard someone say, "My cancer was a blessing?" Well, this is what they were talking about. Through their pain, they learned a lesson that profoundly changed their life.

Ask yourself this question whenever you feel a charge around something. Am I feeling fear, anger, or sadness? Then listen. The first answer that comes to you is the predominant emotion. Next, observe the emotion without judgment. Zoom out to 60,000 feet in the air and just look at it. Resist labeling it. You're going to want to label it good or bad because this is how we've been taught. This is when you begin to reprogram yourself and realize that what it's called is the monkey mind playing games with you. You are the one that chooses how you're going to feel, and how you're going to react. When you feel, you can look at it, and when you recognize what it is, make the choice of how to feel about it. Some people do this easily; for others, it takes practice. You're going to listen, you're going to observe, you're going to tune in to the feelings that are in your body, and the feelings, words, and stories that are coming into your head. You're going to observe. Observe doesn't mean work it out. We're used to being problem solvers. There are some situations and problems that don't require us to intervene for them to be solved. What is amazing in this moment is that the solutions that come out of nowhere – out of the universe – tend to be much more elegant than anything our logical mind could have dreamed.

One of my favorite personal growth authors and teachers, Byron Katie, has a simple process, called Inquiry. I'm going to tell you about one step of that process. There's one piece and one profound question in this process that you need to know. The question is, "Is it true?" The follow-up question is, "Do you absolutely know that it's true?"

Here's the ninja secret sauce of getting through anything quickly and easily. This is something I learned from my other coach, Dan Sullivan, who is a coach to super entrepreneurs. Ask "Who?" not "How?" when you have a problem. Find out Who can help you solve it, not How to solve it. Those of us who were used to problem-solving think that we personally always have to come up with the answer, but the shortcut to getting to the answer is figuring out Who, then going to that person and bringing them into your team in some way.

Here's where you need to check yourself. If you're one of those people who thinks that you have to do everything, and that only you can do it right, and there's nobody else who has more expertise in any area than you, this may be your addiction. Look right square at it and figure out why you feel that way. What do you fear will happen if you enlist the Who, rather than doing it yourself?

My wish for you is that you get results as quickly as possible, rather than having you stumble and fall by going on Doctor Google, or trying to figure it out yourself, or thinking that no one has been down this road before. If I know a shortcut, I'm going to give you the shortcut, and in this chapter, the shortcut is to ask yourself a question, get the answer from your right brain, and identify one of the three emotions causing you consternation and the situation attached to it. Identify the lesson learned from the challenge, and figure out how to have gratitude, love, or joy because of what you learned. Last, find the Who that can help you get results, and don't look for How to do it so you can tough it out alone (the ninja secret sauce shortcut).

Chapter 10

YOU HAVE A "FIX IT" PROTOCOL IN YOU

I want you out of that and to have a fabulous, abundant life. That's why I'm going to teach you how to create your passion protocol. Do it quickly as we're going through the exercises. Flow into it.

I've heard so many stories about hundreds and thousands of dollars of debt, time spent, and sacrifices made, including your family and your friends. The misery behind the beginning of this book and the beginning of my protocol was to get you to a place of calm and clarity, where you can begin to create again. This is the part of the book where you create something for yourself that you can offer to the world. This is your passion protocol. What is it that you can teach in five modules (five steps, forty-five minutes) that are the juicy nuggets you've learned from your years of experience, and that you're going to boil down into a process that you can teach people?

I'm saying this upfront. The further you get away from the medical, the better. Why? Because that is what people are craving. Other stuff. They have tried all the medical stuff. Now they want the "soft" stuff. Tips that work, like what you have been learning, except for their particular pain point. Notice how, as you were doing what is in this book, your life is improving as you have been implementing. Notice how little anyone talks about these things in a medical setting. You've learned some stuff you can take away to teach others, based on your passions or your experiences.

I'm going to give you a model for a typical person walking into a healthcare environment, but remember, you can use the same strategy to create something unrelated to health and offer it up. You can also take those principles that relate to health and teach them anywhere, and from anywhere, so that your life is freer. Because your offering will be unique, you will be paid outside of the system in an ethical way. I'll talk more about that in the next chapter.

Let's say you're an OB-GYN and you have multiple women who come to you because they've been struggling to get pregnant. You've been successful at helping patients conceive, and you have all the pictures on the wall of the people that you've been able to help without them going through expensive, time-consuming, and painful fertility treatments. You've also saved them a lot of heartaches. What was it that you showed them that allowed them to become fertile? Put yourself in the role of the teacher. But you're not teaching adult women; you're teaching eight-year-olds. What are you teaching people to give them satisfaction, and get them started up quick? How can you make it so that they can implement it and see results in a short time? You give them a process where they can see some type of result.

Here's how you put it together. Here's the exact formula, here's what you've been waiting for:

- Module One – quick start guide and what to expect.
- Module Two – foundational information about the underlying condition, specifically laying out common issues and one solution that they can go home and implement.
- Module Three – Emotional components.
- Module Four – You are what you eat or don't eat.
- Module Five – Other Natural Nuggets – supplements, oils, complementary therapies. What else can they do to help themselves?
- Module Six – Success Stories and Party and Awards – And taking it further.

In Module 1, it is important to document where they are in some form or fashion. The easiest way is a one to ten scale. Documenting their emotions of fear, anger, and sadness on that scale is helpful. You will see why in a few modules. Next, have them document where they want to go in the time that is allotted and make sure the goals are realistic. You can present what realistic goals are and have them pick. The end of this class is the most important part – having them visualize their success in a lot of detail. Use the five areas of their life and have them visualize and talk about how all those areas will be positively impacted. Leave every module on a high note and a wrap-up, so they know what to do. Hint: K.I.S.S. – please keep it simple, or you are inviting a failure that you will call non-compliance. You want them to experience success quickly. It is also important in this module to have them agree to keep their promise to themselves and for them to understand about habits, that it takes three weeks to form or break a habit, and about six weeks for the brain to develop the new grooves, new gyri and sulci. New habits are etched into the brain and become part of you in this physical way.

In Module two – Start with asking what good things happened since the last module. Find out what result they got with just a tiny bit of information. This is for you and them. This reinforces that you are awesome and shows them how much control they have over their results. Many times, this is a fun time because people's lives can improve overnight. This happens, especially in groups in which there is a sense of not letting their peers down, which is much more powerful than them letting you down in private.

Focus on the top three physical signs or symptoms of your selected condition. Why three? Because three is simple and digestible in a forty-five-minute module. Always keep in mind that what most people want is relief from their pain and control and independence. Your teachings are designed to help them overcome in a way that they can do on their own. This is where you teach them the nuggets that aren't easily found on Google. Leave time to answer questions and problems, and let the magic happen when members of the group coach each other.

Module Three is all about emotions. Do a positive emotions assessment in this session on a scale from one to ten. That is why I gave you the simple six emotions. Whatever condition you are teaching about has its own emotional footprint in every patient. Allowing people to talk about their emotions and listening is therapeutic. This isn't a counseling session, and you must limit the time by using a timer and adhering to the rules. Strictly. You don't want someone hijacking the session and bringing down the energy. Start with the three health-harming emotions and talk about stress and what happens in the body. Simplified. To wrap it up, focus on the health-promoting emotions and have them pick one, only one, that they can implement for the next week.

Module Four is about lifestyle. In every single condition, there are foods that help it and foods that make it worse. Ask them what food they believe will help or hurt. Think again in threes. Give them three of each, and directions on how to buy it, how to prepare it, and ways to get it easily. Anything you ask people to stop doing, think. Talk to them about knowing themselves and if weaning or cold turkey is best for them. Also talk to them about any emotions surrounding letting go, or fears about letting go of a particular food that is harming them. Notice you have dealt with the emotions before you deal with these lifestyle issues. Why? Because they have to understand that stress affects everything, and you want to get them to a positive emotional state so that whatever you give them as far as a lifestyle change will work and stick.

Module Five is about Other helpful tips and modalities. At this point, depending on how far apart you are spacing the sessions, they should be at least one month in or three to four months in, if you are doing monthly modules (spacing of one to two weeks is great because it forces people to do and make changes quickly). Talking about those areas that patients love to do on their own is ideal in this module, like supplements, which include vitamins, minerals, herbs, homeopathic medicine, and the like. Also, complementary modalities offered by other professionals that work. You are giving them permission to help themselves and also share with you what they are doing. This also is about helping them streamline and simplify. Remember to assess at the beginning of the teaching what positive change they had since the last module.

Module Six is meant to celebrate and talk about next steps and taking it further. Whether you are doing this in person or online, plan a celebration. If they are virtual, send out what you want them to bring to class – some type of treat to reward their success. In the beginning, after hearing their successes, you are going to tell them what the next steps would be for them to get results. Now here is the thing. Most of them will have gotten a result, but not fully. You need them to understand that the magic number is 100. It takes about 100 days for a significant change that is lasting. You want to invite them to the next phase of at least three months. At this point, they have gotten results, and it is fun for you and them. You must always guide them to what is next.

Now what if you have decided at this point, I can't be bothered with patients. As I said before, put together the five-step process to guide someone through and teach them. Intellectual property is what people want. You can help them solve a problem that they want to learn, like how to play the piano. Do you say it cannot be learned in five weeks? Of course not, but you can get them started, and with some success using your particular process, you can teach them virtually.

Just as I am guiding you through this book, look back and notice my step by step unique process to get you creating yourself and your brand in a different way. Besides using this process with doctors and other healthcare practitioners, I have helped entrepreneurs in other areas.

An entrepreneur who was a pharmacist worked with me in one of my VIP days. He had developed a unique non-pharmacologic formula that works to get rid of pain. One of the unique qualities about his formulation is that it works on the emotional response to pain. He was having trouble getting people to understand how his formulation worked. We came up with The Get Rid of Your Pain Matrix, in which he would explain the five components of pain and what causes them and how to solve each of the components. One of the components of pain is the emotional response and the solution to changing that is – you guessed it – his product. His product with the entire protocol is very powerful in getting people out of pain, thus we have The Get Rid of Your Pain Matrix.

I guided a LinkedIn specialist to put together his process of using LinkedIn to turn contacts into clients. The LinkedIn Profit Blueprint we developed has six parts, which guide on do's and don'ts of using LinkedIn effectively, which include profile graphics, profile wording, outreach, invitations, posting, and messaging. We broke down to a formula what he does for his clients so that he could easily tell you what result he guided his clients to.

When you work on this, have fun. The more fun you have while creating, the better it will come across when you tell someone about it. One of the most fun things I do with my entrepreneur and physician clients is to take them through my creative process and dive deep into the areas where they get stuck so they can quickly get around the obstacle that is holding them back. This area of seeing your own unique process can be difficult because when you start doing it, you are so close in that you can't see it. You are in the forest and can only see the trunks of the trees. When I coach, I am in the airplane looking down over your forest and can ask questions about what is going on in the forest so you can lay out the important aspects in a way that allows you to become a master teacher. You already have the knowledge to be the master teacher, but no one has taught you how to teach in an engaging way that sets you apart.

As you create, keep in mind The Group Visit Launch Formula, The Get Rid of Your Pain Matrix, and The LinkedIn Profit Blueprint, along with my Too Smart to Be Struggling Reboot that I have been leading you through. The secret is to break it down to simplicity rather than throwing everything together with every tiny detail that it becomes overwhelming. Just like I have been taking you by the hand, and just like I take my clients by the hand, I want you create so that you could teach your concepts to a twelve-year-old and they will get it and be able to implement whatever you are teaching.

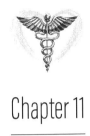

Chapter 11

GET MORE MONEY WITHOUT WORKING MORE HOURS

Many doctors are unhappy with their financial situation. It's understandable to have a lot of debt and feel like you have no way to pay it. You feel like, with your current position, you are wearing golden handcuffs. You have to do it. You may be paid well, you may be not paid well, but you feel like that you have to be in this position because you have no other choice. You've never been taught how to do business, or exactly how to make money, other than going out and getting a job. Period.

First thing I want to address is that, in the last chapter, I gave you a framework for creating your intellectual property, whether that is something that has to do with medicine and health care, or something completely different. I wanted to give you a framework so that you're still thinking about it, and know that this is how money is made. Let me address something else. Everyone has beliefs about money, and also a set point of how much money they can have and earn. What do I mean by that? I have assessed in people the belief system that keeps them from earning money, the amount of money that they want, and the amount of money that they need. Usually, these beliefs are set way back in childhood, based on your familial situation. You have ideas about how money is made. Let me give you an example. This is from my particular background, and reading and understanding of something that I realized when I was a Sunday school teacher teaching people in my church how to live financially according to biblical principles. There's a passage in the Bible about money that is often misquoted. The passage states, "The love of money is a root of evil." The common misquote is, "Money is the root of evil."

I'm pointing out what the passage says versus the misquote of it because this has to do with the belief system. People misquote the passage because of their own belief that money is evil. Are you one of those people who feels that money is evil? If the answer to that is yes, this may be one of the reasons that you are having a hard time earning money, and so I'm going to talk a little bit about belief systems and money later on. But I want you to begin to examine your belief system surrounding money, and understand that this informs how much money you can make, and how much money you can receive, and what you feel money's meaning is or is not.

People have a particular belief system about how money is earned and doctors, in particular, think they only deserve money when they work hard. It might be something that has been taught in their home, or they've learned it just from going through their life.

My client Melanie, a well-decorated physician with lots of certificates and experience, shared with me that one of her beliefs about life in general, back to her childhood, is that you have to take the hard route. She confided in me that she remembers judging her siblings and classmates in elementary school. "They're taking the easy route. I'm not going to take the easy route. I'm going to work hard and do the hardest thing I can think of. They're lazy, but not me. I work hard." In everything that she's done, it's been hard and complicated, including earning. Does this ring a bell with you? Do you believe that, if it's not hard, it somehow must not be worth it? That smart people do the hard things and dummies take the easy way?

Your career and earning money don't have to be hard. They can be easy, and feel easy to you, be extraordinarily helpful and transformative for you and the people you serve. I hope this is a revelation for you, and you start asking yourself in everything you do – how can I make this easy and simple? In some people, this belief system can be changed easily. In fact, I had a client, Carol, who, in only one session, was able to let go of the "life is hard" belief, and next day, was able to make more money.

From working with many clients, I noticed certain patterns surrounding money. These patterns even manifested in their health in interesting ways. With doctors and other healthcare practitioners, limiting beliefs surrounding money can not only keep your income lower than you like, but also block the results you are getting with your clients. I call the characteristic in a person's energy field that surrounds money and finances, the Earning Energy Imprint™. Everyone has an Earning Energy Imprint. When you assess your financial situation and consider your net worth, you can see where your EEI is. When you learn how to raise your earning energy, you can raise the amount of money that is going to come into your life and stay in your life.

Let's begin to raise your earning energy right now. This is why I gave you a framework in the last chapter on how to package your intellectual property.

I want to encourage you to offer your services at a high value. You are valuable. If you are not earning enough, it's because you have decided that you are not valuable and you don't deserve it. Now, one of my coaches, Lisa Sasavitch, talks about one's "having" level. What is your "having" level? Your "having" level means how much money you can accept at this time. Think about how much money you've ever gotten at one time, and how much you believe you should charge for your services. How much money has ever been in your possession or your bank account?

My having level has allowed me to get into seven figures. A lot of doctors have been used to being in six figures, some in the low six figures, and some in the five-figure mark. That is a problem when you are in a lot of debt. I read about a doctor who was distressed over being $350,000 in debt. Wow, that's a lot. In order to get rid of $350,000 of debt, you're going to need to bring in a significant amount of income. Well, how do you do that? You're not going to do it by earning in the low four or five figures, or even in the low six figures. You're probably not going to be able to even enjoy your life when you have to pay back $350,000 of debt in student loans, plus a house, plus your car, plus your living expenses, plus your food, plus your family. Your income needs to be a lot higher. Let's talk about how much you think you can have, and how much you deserve. I often hear doctors talk about how much they charge per hour. That's the idea of trading time for money. You know that visits are $150 or $200. Now, one of the horrible things that doctors have accepted is that their value is what the insurance companies will pay them, and they think there's no other way.

There is another way. Here it is. You can let go of the insurance system, and you can bundle your services and offer them to people at a value they will pay for.

Let me give you an example. All through your life, or at least, your professional life, you have been buying quite expensive bundled services. Number one is college. Number two, medical school. Number three, continuing medical education. Number four, certification programs. All of these are bundled services, where they set the semester cost.

Let's say a semester costs $525,000. You paid it. It was a bundled service, and you didn't even think about questioning what that service was. The understanding was that, at the end of it, you would have what you wanted. A college degree, which could get you into medical school, which could get you into residency, which could get you into fellowship, which could get you into the job that you thought that you wanted. Your bliss was the prospect being hired for your dream position using your newly acquired knowledge (not even a guarantee or even help in finding a job). You were given what you felt that you wanted. The transformation was a medical degree, a certificate in functional medicine, a certification in thyroid disease. This was a bundled program. You paid a lot for that bundled program. You are going to do the same with your services. Now think about it.

You're saying, "How can I do that? That's a big college, that's a big medical school, they've been there for years, and everybody knows it." Well, people come out every day with these kinds of products and services in bundles. Let me break it down simply. I'm going to use something that you might say yuck to, but it's the best simple example. You are running around, and you haven't eaten. You don't have a lot of time. You drive up to the fast food window. What do you see on the menu? You see bundles (or combos, to use fast food lingo). You see burgers, fries, and a drink, packaged together at one price. Every fast food restaurant has that. When they put it all together, it tends to be priced less than each individual product added together. You're going to do the same thing with your services. You're going to offer to people burgers, fries, and a drink all together, except your burgers, fries, and drinks are the pieces of your intellectual property. How do you value your intellectual property? Any way that you want to, but I'll give you some suggestions a little bit later on. Here's a piece that you need to grasp about your particular having level, and your particular investment. Right now, you're going to offer someone your intellectual property separately. I want to ask you, as you're going forward, besides your schooling, have you ever invested in yourself at a high level?

If the answer to that is no, that you have not invested in yourself at the high level, you or your energy is going to be such that people aren't going to be able to give that to you.

Think about it. Have you ever invested in a program for someone's intellectual property? A program that, at the end, would be giving you something you wanted? And you paid $2,000, or $5,000, $25,000, $50,000, $100,000? Have you ever made a type of investment in yourself, in something that was intellectual property, that didn't have a certificate, at the end of it?

Yes or no?

Once you do that for yourself once – decide that you deserve whatever it is that you can invest in, outside of the formal education system – you'll be on your way.

For instance, I have been in a business Mastermind where the price ticket was $55,000. I have been in a business Master-mind where the price was at $1,000. I invested in myself and my business, outside of medical college training and certifications, in someone else's intellectual property up to $88,000 at this point.

You're saying, "Oh, my God, how could you do that?" Because they bundled my bliss. They were offering to me the intellectual property to help me bundle the bliss and give myself a raise.

By now, you're looking at this and saying, "How can I ask for that?" Well, you're going to determine how much you've invested in yourself up until now, and you're going to consider going somewhere and investing in yourself by learning other skills to be able to bundle your bliss.

You need to invest in yourself. You need to decide that it's worth it. You deserve it. One of the biggest reasons to make a big investment in yourself and into somebody else's intellectual property is so that you do not feel like a fraud asking for the money for your products or services. The biggest way to have the wrong energy in presenting your products and services is to have never done it yourself, because the energy that you are putting out is "I would never spend this kind of money on myself" while you're asking someone else to spend that type of money. If you're wondering why people are only spending certain amounts of money on you, it's likely because, in that same area, you've never spent more than that type of money on yourself. In order to get results, you first have to go out and make the investment in yourself, somewhere in some area.

I would recommend that you look at your area of health. You are a doctor, a healthcare practitioner, and you're talking about health. Health means being well first, but have you invested money in being well? It's incongruent, if you are sick and you are offering health to someone else. Think about that. These are concepts that maybe you have never thought about, and these are concepts that are not what medical school teaches you. But they are so important to how the universe works, and how you're going to get what you deserve.

At this point in time, you are already getting what you deserve, and if you don't like what that is, you need a system to change it. The system to change it isn't going to be to get another certification. The system to change it is different. Remember the Einstein statement about insanity being to do the same thing over and over and expecting a different result? Up to this point, you might have only invested in getting knowledge, but you've not invested in how to create money, how to create wealth, or how to create programs.

You must invest time and money in your own health. You may not have invested in being well, and so invest in being well yourself, and all of a sudden, once you make that investment, you're going to notice that even in your practice with your patients, your clients are going to start to do better in their own bodies and that means they are going to start to heal simply because you have shifted your energy.

How can that be? Do it for a good six months to do your own trial. Again you are your own case study. Test out this concept so you can see for yourself what happens. Do It. Invest in yourself and your health. Whatever you are suffering from right now, go to someone who has a program that is different from what you know or understand from your training. Go to someone who has a program that says, "I can help you with your condition and I'm going to guide you to get you better," and go for it. But also, go for it with a mindset that it's going to work. Invest in your colleague, and their knowledge that they are a master at what they are doing to be able to help you.

You should understand that every day, people pay for these types of products and services. Think about it. You've gone out and you've asked people at times to build your website. Or, do your social media or some other product or service that is intellectual property. Somebody might have quoted to you $1,520, or $25,000 to build your website, and somebody else might have quoted to you $5,000 or even $1,500 dollars to build your website. Now, how much does it cost to build a website? Nobody knows what it costs. The price has to do with what that person or company has decided that it's worth, and that you, in your mind, have justified, based on what you're going to get from it. you decide to pay whatever it is, but who's to say whether a website is worth $1,500 dollars or $50,000?

You can do the same thing.

Now, you're probably saying you don't know anybody who would spend $2,000, $5,000, $50,000, $100,000 for intellectual property, but look all around you. There are people like that. Ask people if they have ever done something like that. If you've ever paid a consultant or coach, you've probably spent that amount of money to get a result. You are going to offer people results. Not features, but results. If you think that the patients around you cannot make that investment, you are likely wrong. Change your belief system. Now, let me give you some examples. You're going to look around you, and suddenly see that even your patients on Medicaid have thousand-dollar smartphones.

I remember, back in my practice, I had a full-service eye care practice, which meant that not only did I offer medical services, there were other services I offered that people could pay for out of pocket. Think contact lenses and glasses. Now contact lenses are a commodity. It's hard to charge a lot, because people can order them over the internet. You're pretty limited on what you can charge for contact lenses. However, glasses are different. Think about glasses. There's all different kinds of frames. There are cheap frames, there are expensive designer frames. There's junk. There's Gucci and Dior, and all those designers that you know so well. You see people walking around with Ray Bans every single day. Look at your glasses. You may have glasses with no logo, or you may have glasses with a logo. You paid a lot of money simply to show that logo.

How much was that logo worth? Was it worth $500? $750? $1,000? Yes, frames for prescription glasses and sunglasses can go up into the thousands of dollars. Why? Because they're stylish, and they have a logo – that, you know – but is the plastic or the metal that they're made of worth that cost?

In my office in my dispensary, I would observe that even people who you would expect had limited funds would spend generously on themselves. This was back at the time when I accepted Medicaid. I had a gentleman, Jerry, who drove up in his Mercedes Benz, and presented his Medicaid card to our office. He wore a stylish suit with the latest cut dress pants, designer shoes, and haute couture glasses. I did his eye exam. I was paid $22 for his eye exam.

I walked him into my optical dispensary with his prescription and said, you can take a look here. Now, at that point, I had a Medicaid selection frames, but the Medicaid were in no uncertain terms butt-ugly. Yucky. You would not want to be seen in them.

If you have extra money and you want to look good, you will not buy those Medicaid frames, you'll buy something else. I had all levels of different types of frames in my optical dispensary, from Medicaid up to designer frames.

What did Jerry pick? He picked the $750 Gucci frames with the progressive Luxe lenses that are transitions, with the reflective coating on them. I'm telling you, this gentleman picked out a pair of glasses that, by the time he added on all the benefits that he wanted, cost $1,500. He looked good. He had transition lenses that got dark outside and got light inside. They had anti-reflective coating, glare protection, progressive lenses (so there was no line). He could see the road while driving, and he could glance at his smartphone and see all that for $1,500.

Jerry could have bought all the non-name brand stuff which my optical dispensary also offered, but he chose to go the high end. He could have gotten the free glasses that his

Medicaid would cover with no out of pocket costs for him. Jerry bought the $1,500 glasses. Why? Jerry knows and deeply believes that he deserves it.

He didn't want to pay for his medical care. That wasn't worth it to him to spend money on. He presented his Medicaid card for the exam. What was valuable to Jerry was his image, and he was willing to spend the money that he had on his image. I was compensated $22 for the eye exam, and $1,500 – fifty percent of which was profit to my business.

I want you to think about this. Every day, you're around people who make those same types of buying decisions. This is why I told you to just look around at people's iPhones or iPads or smartphones or whatever they walk around with. Look at the pocketbooks. Look at the shoes. Look at the cars that people are driving.

Practically everybody, no matter what their financial status is, has decided that they deserve some product that is expensive.

Why is that? Many times, it's because that product was packaged or branded. I want you to package and brand yourself. This is why I had you create your image of looking good, because people buy people, and people buy brands, and people buy transformation.

The transformation for Jerry with those glasses is the image of just being it and there. Nobody knew that he carried a Medicaid card in his wallet. When they looked at him, he had all outward items of success. The car, the phone. The shoes and the glasses.

what are some of the things that will help you charge for your products and services? First, think about taking it out of a particular medical realm.

Let's talk about putting together your intellectual property. You bundle it, and you value it however you want. But let me give you some easy numbers to use. Let's say you're going to offer your program in four or five or six modules, and, since you're working now, you want to offer it online an hour at a time. A lot of people regularly, every day, pay about $2,000 for those type of programs.

If you do it online, you can offer your services to a group of people, and ask them each to pay $2,000. Five sessions in your office, if you're charging hourly at $150 to $200 – five times two, that's about $1,000. Well, what I'm saying is, if you can offer five sessions to a group of people, and charge them $2,000 each, you're not going to be using an hourly type rate. That's not how you think about it, you think about the transformation that you're going to offer people. What is the transformation? How are they going to feel and be different after you guide them to what they want?

When Jerry bought the glasses, it wasn't about the plastic in the frame or the plastic in the lens. It was about how it made him feel. It made him feel successful. It made him feel stylish. That was something that was quite important to him. Your people around you are going to pay you for a solution to get out of their trouble. What is the solution that you're offering to do that?

One of the things is to name your program, or offer a solution. Think about even using the word "solution" in the name of it. Let's talk about the elements of a strong name.

One of the first elements is using the word "the" in front of whatever it is.

This is important because when you use "the," it denotes that it is THE One. THE Only, it's THE solution to your problem.

The solution to the problem. Another way to think of the first word or words in the name of your product is to put your name in front of it.

For example Dr Veronica's Rejuvenation Journey or The Rejuvenation Journey.

It's yours, it's nobody else's, you created it. "The" rejuvenation journey means, it is not one, not somebody else's. It's not just rejuvenation journey, it's not just any rejuvenation journey. It is the one and only. This is important for the emotion and psychology behind it, it's either yours, with your name on it, it's important, and, especially if you're putting the doctor in front of it, because doctors still denote something special, because everybody can get it. Dr Veronica's Rejuvenation Journey, or The Rejuvenation Journey is something that's important. Think about naming your program with the first words of your name with the doctor or the word.

And at the end of it, is something like a word that shows them that this is the answer. Try out Solution, Roadmap, Blueprint, Program. Matrix. Protocol. Journey. These are some of the words that you can use at the end.

What do you put in the middle? After "The" or "Your Name" and before the end anchor word?

You put in the middle between those two words the result or the purpose that your signature protocol delivers. Think about what they are going to get out of it. This is why I named my health transformation program The Rejuvenation Journey, because what are they going to get is rejuvenated.

I have a program called The Group Visit Launch Formula. At the beginning of the name is what they want to learn how to do. This is the formula for practitioners who would like to start seeing their clients. They want to learn how to do integrate group visits into their practice quickly and easily. Where do you start and how do you start? That is the launch. Voila. The Group Visit Launch Formula.

Think about naming your program like this as you follow along my real-life example. "The" or "your name" on the front. What you will give to them in the middle. At the end, what is it. It's a launch. It's a formula.

It's a system that allows you to bundle their bliss. What the name does is it specifically tells them what they're going to get. The importance of packaging your services like that, with modules and with a name, and with the transformation that you are going to give them, is all about having it so that there is a value there, the value creation, and there's nothing else that they can compare it to. Is there another Group Visit Launch Formula out there? Well, maybe, but I haven't seen it, and what is the Group Visit Launch Formula? I give the exact formula that I use to launch successful group programs. I tell you, do this, do that, do this, do that, and at the end of it, you're going to have your group program. I've been giving you bits and pieces in this chapter. But if you just want to look at one little thing, the Group Visit Launch Formula and go through those steps, it's the best way to strip out everything else and talk about it.

I talk about exactly how to do it, and more of the logistics in it, including marketing, and how to decide what your program is going to be. Easy ways to think about it. That's what I talk about in the Group Visit Launch Formula. By the end, everyone has their own group visit program. While they were in the program, they were doing the work on the way to the launch, so that by the time they get to the end, five to six weeks later, they can launch their program because they've already been marketing and advertising it.

That's the type of service that you are going to offer to people – services that are valuable and you can offer alongside your insurance-based practice. Or you can take it outside, and offer it separately. You could start a new business with your previous skills, where you package them in a different way. Or with a new skill, which is why I wanted you to look at all the different things that you have been good at in your life, or that you have a passion for, because it's important. You're going to teach well what you have a real passion for. That's why I teach well about group visits, because I have a passion for teaching, and I realized this is a way of teaching that I have learned and taught other people, and that has been extraordinarily fun and successful. I have a passion for it, because I've seen it transform the lives of my clients. Also, and this is the most wonderful thing, imagine when you bring together a group of people, and they heal all together. They have results all together; they feel good all together. That allowed me to go back to feeling like I am doing what I originally set out to do when I wanted to be a doctor as a four-year-old. It allowed me to be able to help people heal again, and that is the best feeling in the world. Even better, they invested in themselves, and they were happy to invest in themselves, because I gave them the solution to their problem. They bought the solution to their problem with their hard-earned dollars.

Let me address another concept. When you are not offering your products and services in this way, you are blocking the healing of other people. You are blocking other people's happiness and success. You have to give people the opportunity to decide that they deserve to have what you're giving to them. To decide they want to demonstrate to the universe, with their hard-earned dollars, that they value themselves enough to pay for a product or service that's going to help them. If you don't offer them the opportunity to do that, you block their success.

It works the same for everyone. This is a principle that a lot of people have never heard about – earning an inner money. Money is simply a form of energy that people use to exchange for a product or service and get something. How you spend your money shows exactly what you value in life. There are a lot of people who will spend their money on a smartphone, and they don't spend their money on their health. Guess what? They're sick. There's other people who decide, "I'm going to invest in myself, and my health is so important to me that I'm going to figure out a way to pay for it." People make these decisions every day. You may have made the decision to invest. I know you've made the decisions to invest in learning how to be a doctor, but maybe you've never invested in your particular health, if you are ill now or struggling now. Maybe it's time to go to a practitioner that can help you get a result, and pay them, make the energetic exchange – the money exchange – to show the universe that you value your health. Now isn't that a revolutionary idea!

I'm telling you, if you want people to pay you for your products and services, especially if you're offering health services, go pay somebody else and show that other practitioner that they are valued like you want to be valued.

Here is what you must grasp. When you are paying for a product or service, what is your feeling when you're doing it? What are you thinking? What emotion? What was your feeling when you went out and bought your smartphone? Didn't you feel thrilled when you were making that purchase? When you were taking on the debt to go to medical school, what was the feeling behind it? Was it gratitude that you got into medical school, and you were glad there was a loan program to allow you to pursue your dream? Was it joy because you were starting down the road to be able to save the world with the gifts and talents you would be developing in your training? You were so in love with going into medicine that you willingly paid thousands of dollars or took on thousands of dollars of debt – without any guarantee of a future position or promise of how much you would be able to earn.

When you drive off in the car you bought or the house you stepped in, even if it is an apartment you don't own, you probably did it with a positive feeling. Gratitude and joy.

You're happy that you have found a car you want to buy – that Honda, that Toyota, the Mercedes Benz – and maybe you haven't gotten there yet, but you have been looking through the pages of wanting to have the car of your dreams. What does that make you feel like? You feel joyful riding in it. When it's time, and you have the money to be able to go buy it, you're feeling joy. Whenever you make a purchase of anything, including your personal growth and spiritual development, how you feel sends a message to the Universe.

A lot of people spend money with the negative emotions of fear, anger and resentment, or grief. You're sending a message to the Universe that this is how you feel about money. Are you spending money with fear? "Oh, my God! Oh, my God! Oh! I don't know how I'm gonna pay this." Are you spending money with grief? "I hate spending money on anything. It makes me so sad I have to give away my money, I hate giving away my money." Are you stingy, or you're stingy because you're fearful that there's no monetary resources in the universe and no more is going to come to you? Are you an angry spender? Are you angry that you have to pay for your health care? A lot of doctors are angry spenders. This is you, if you have ever gotten mad at another doctor who charges more than you and gets it. Or if you are seriously peeved at doctors or coaches and consultants who offer any kind of high-ticket program that is unattached to an institution, degree, or certificate.

I got a notice in my inbox from Doximity, the social media site for doctors only, with the subject line "Women In Medicine." I opened it and saw a message that was written by a fellow female physician about bad career advice given to women physicians and what they could do about it. After she laid out the advice and some solutions, she offered her retreat for women physicians. I was appalled at the nasty, snarky comments, especially the ones criticizing that she offered a service that was thousands of dollars. Angry public commentary about money. These physicians are sending a message to the Universe that is hurting them, not the doctor who wrote the article to give other doctors the opportunity to invest in themselves.

If you are having trouble getting the money you want, closely examine your money blocking attitudes and emotions. Do you see how it's coming back around again to fear, anger, and sadness?

This may be why you can't make money, because of your money blocks. You've heard about money blocks. You have tricked yourself into the trap that you don't have enough certifications, or your website isn't right, or the hospital administrators who decide the salaries are greedy jerks. That is not what the core of your problem is. Those are distracting pieces of data. Your emotions surrounding spending and receiving money has set your Earning Energy Imprint.

I love to work with people in this area of money. When I have a new offering, and people are not enrolling as I expect, I examine my money energy and beliefs surrounding that program and my worth in offering it. Reading about this is raising your awareness, and a small shifting of your earning energy from fear, anger, and sadness to gratitude, love, and joy in the area of spending. It is a whole new energy opening up for you and money will begin to flow. When you invest in yourself the way you want other people to invest in you, based on faith, that is another big opening.

Spend money and do it gratefully.

I only want to receive money from people who are investing in themselves with gratitude, and who are showing that attitude to the Universe by allowing me to receive this token of their appreciation for sharing my gifts and talent with them to enrich their lives.

I don't want to receive money from people if they're giving it to me in fear, anger or sadness.

When I got the email from my client who had invested over $10K with me, that they were happy and grateful that they had met me, I realized that she allowed me to receive her money and energy, and I allowed her to make the energetic exchange so that she could demonstrate how important is was to her to heal. She invested in herself with gratitude, love, and joy. Note, I had to offer the service. This is step one. People are unable to invest with you if you never make the offer. You have to get it out of your head, open your mouth, tell people you have a service, and tell them how it will help them. You, too, must go out and offer people the service, and give people the opportunity to make the energetic exchange called money, invest in themselves, and do it with gratitude, love, and joy. When someone says yes, they are saying yes to themselves. When someone refuses, they are saying no to themselves. It's not about how good you or I are at our service. It's about how much the other person values themselves, and whether or not they feel they deserve to invest energy (also known as money) in themselves.

In order for them to be able to understand what it is you have to bundle their bliss, you have to put it in words that they can understand, where they can see that the program you're offering is the solution to their pains, and that you are going to walk them through how to solve their pains.

Chapter 12

SEEING YOUR BEST NEXT MOVE

The last step in this process is called The C.A.R.E. Solution. It's The C.A.R.E. Solution, because I always want my clients to remember that they must care for themselves. By naming this The C.A.R.E. Solution, you always see the word "care." It is important that you understand that you are the most good to the world when you can show up the best, and that means you are in the best form. The only way you can be in the best form is to care for yourself first. You might have heard this as it's popular today for people to say it, but not a lot of people know exactly how to do it. In the beginning of this book, in the first step, I told you to create White Space. The reason why I told you to create White Space is because it was a way of forcing you into caring for yourself. But you had to calm down and slow down to be able to do that.

The way to think about everything going forward is to be able to figure out a process that you can go through that will always work. The reason that caring for yourself first is important is because it allows you to have clarity in this area, and that's the first step in The C.A.R.E. Solution. The C is for clarity, clarity in what you want in your life, in what you want your life to look like. After you figure out what you want your life to look like, then it becomes a reverse engineering process. What do I want my life to look like? Here's what I want it to look like. You've already done a lot of work on this, going through this process. Once you know what you want your life to look like, the second step is to ask yourself what career choice you can make to be able to allow your life to look like that. Clarity in what you want for your life will lead to clarity in your career path. It's not just about you wanting to make a certain amount of money. The reason you want to make a certain amount of money is because you want what's called freedom. The freedom, for me, is called the "I don't need your money and I can quit right now" freedom.

That's what I want for you. The "I don't need your money and I can quit right now" freedom. Come with clarity in the area of what exactly you would like your life to look like and a system and formula to achieve freedom with your own unique and branded intellectual property offered as a high-ticket program.

It's a beautiful thing to be able to decide, for every moment of your life, exactly what you want it to be. my goal in this was to show you how to begin to create that. Clarity is the first big C – clarity on what you would like your life to look like in the five areas.

And then, clarity on what will get you to those areas.

Now, as you're creating your life and your business, you're always going to be offering people products or services; you're always going to be convincing people to say yes or no to whatever you want. Think of it with your kids – you have to convince them sometimes to eat something, you have to convince them to come home, you have to convince your wife or your husband or your partner to do what you want to do, and whoever wins is the person who is the best convinced, sir, and with passion.

And it's not always logical at all. How we make decisions is not based on logic. Decision making is emotional even when we trick ourselves into believing how logical we are. Get comfortable with this as a fact of marketing as we go on to the A of the CARE, which is in Avatar Attraction. Who do you want around you? Be clear about who you want around you. It's important that you know exactly what that person looks like. Now I use the word "avatar," because, think of the movie *Avatar.*

Zoe, an avatar, has a particular personality, look, preferences in what she eats and reads and does, likes, dislikes, and a way she makes decisions. That may be your avatar. Imagine when you talk to her, its going to be about how she can maintain her beautiful blue skin and large eyes and what to do in her treehouse in the magical woods. The worlds and language you use are not going to be the same as what you would say to a man in New York City about how to get rid of his acne.

Okay, so the next part of doing any business is not what your specialty is, it's not what your niche is – you're going to decide your niche, it's going to become clear what your niche is when you've decided what you want for your life. It's even deeper than that. It's not that you're a cardiologist or a endocrinologist or an ophthalmologist or a family practitioner. That's your area of specialty; that's your little niche, but who in those areas, are you set aside to work with specially? Are you a master at maintaining the beauty and texture of blue skin in the rainforest of Zoe's and her women friends? Or are you simply a dermatologist that treats skin rashes?

Who do you want to work with? Who do you like to work with, and who are the people in which you get the best results? I had to go through that exercise, because it gives you a picture of exactly who you like to work with, even if it's teaching the piano. If that brings you passion and joy, do you want to play the piano all day? And do you want to teach other people to play the piano? Who is it that's going to be your avatar for that? Here's a good example:

Because my husband's primary language is French, (and his family lives in France), I decided that I wanted to be able to speak and understand French when I go to France.

I stumbled and bumbled around to figure out exactly what was going to work for me to learn French. First, I tried Rosetta Stone. It didn't work.

Next, I tried Duolingo and other apps. They didn't work. My French had zero improvement.

Next, I went to a site called TakeLessons. I looked there for teachers, but I had no idea how to select a teacher. They all kind of looked the same to me. Well, they had reviews, so I read the reviews. I looked at the reviews, and I picked a teacher. I took some French classes a couple times a week for a few months. But I realized I wasn't learning anything. I wasn't getting how to make a sentence. I couldn't remember how to conjugate the verbs, the homework wasn't helpful to me, it just wasn't clicking for me. I knew I wasn't going to learn to speak French this way, and how did I know this? When I went to France after taking six months of lessons, I felt like I was in the exact same place I was when I had been in France before I had taken lessons at all. I decided this wasn't working for me.

I went to an entrepreneurial event, and as I networked with other participants at this event, I told them I was actively seeking a new French teacher. I had a speakers spot on stage at this event, and part of my presentation highlighted my quest to learn to speak French.

Well, as the universe would have it, all of a sudden, a woman steps up to the mic and says, "Hi, my name is Angelique, and I'm a French teacher." She goes on to ask a question about her business to the host of the event.

Can you believe it? I'm at entrepreneurial event. Up to the mic walks a French teacher. I've only met one other language teacher in my ten years on the entrepreneur's circle of events. There were hundreds of people at this particular event. I'm wondering, how am I going to find that lady? I got a good look at her from across the room and barely remember what she looks like, and there's so many people here.

By the end of the event, I was sitting and talking to someone, forgetting that I said I wanted to meet the French teacher, and in walks Angelique. she said to me, "Someone told me that you were looking for me."

I said, "Oh, my God, I'm so happy that you came over and found me. I need a French teacher. Can I talk to you?" And thus, begin my relationship with Angelique, who spurred me to do an French immersion program, and has become one of my good friends. We discuss our business together, and she teaches French, and I help her with getting clarity in her business. It's wonderful. I made a new friend and have someone to talk to about our businesses together.

In talking to Angelique, we talked about the type of people she likes to teach to speak French. Well guess what? I am her avatar.

She teaches almost exclusively and wants an educated, motivated, mid-life high performing professional woman who enjoys and perseveres through new challenges, who wants to learn French to increase her life experiences, and wants to become proficient enough so that she can live and/or work in France or in a French-speaking community.

I am the perfect avatar for Angelique.

When you are thinking about who it is that you are going to offer your products and services to, think about Zoe in the movie *Avatar* or Angelique and what makes me her perfect French student.

Just a side note about my French.

One of the best things that you can do to keep your brain working well is to take on a new and different and challenging learning experience. We know from research that this is how you form new neural connections.

At the top of the list to form new neural connections and prevent mushy brain, or in medical terminology, cognitive decline of which Alzheimer's poster child for, is to learn and/ or master a foreign language. Learning French has been one of the most challenging endeavors that I have taken up. I didn't want to just learn French, to be able to get an A on the test. I want to learn French, so that I can enjoy being with family and friends while in France, and I love the opportunity to live or work in a French environment.

After working with Angelique for ten months, I decided to go to an immersion program in France at L'Institut de Français for four weeks.

Eight and a half hours a day, four days a week.

When you walk into the gates of L'Institut de Francias, only French is allowed from day two (day one is orientation in English). You eat breakfast speaking French; you have lunch speaking French with the professors dining with you. Tours around town during the first week are done one sentence in French and then the same sentence in French.

What a scary experience. What an exhilarating experience.

I went from Debutante Deux to Intermediate in four weeks. Angelique had taught me enough French so that I was not Debutante Une. One Friday of week three, it was my turn to do an exposé – sit in front of the class and present about me for at least ten minutes, all in French, and to take questions in French from my fellow students and professor. I spoke for thirty minutes. I couldn't believe it myself. I was able to talk about my life, my profession, my children, my husband and his family and my hobbies – all in French.

I'm one of the avatars of L'Institut de Francais. Their main avatar? Diplomat types that are going to live in a French speaking country and must master French at a high enough level to speak, read, and write to represent their country's interest. They also cater to other high-performing professionals there who are learning French as a hobby. Their hobby is to be able to master another language. There were seven other doctors in the program. There was a judge. There was the director of security for the country of Norway and a diplomat from Singapore. A socialite from Colombia. A lady who opened 1400

Zahra boutiques around the world. A Russian lawyer who is an expert in real estate. That's just a few of the interesting people who were in my classes and became my friends.

I'm telling you this so that you start thinking about different types of people who might be your avatar. What you might say to them to attract them. What you might say to them to convince them to take advantage of your offering. When I say convince, it's more of an attraction than a chasing.

When you know the best type of person you can help and get results, you're able to demonstrate that you can get a result for them.

The people who are right will find you. You're going to put yourself out there in a particular way so you are "find-able." People will begin to find you.

Revenue money. We've talked a little bit about money. We've talked a lot about money. It's always on your mind. Eighty percent of your day is spent in either money-making activities or thinking about money.

Revenue is important. Profits are important. It's going to allow you to move forward; however, you want to have your revenue come to you in a particular way that works for you. Flowing because what you are doing is easy to you. It can be easy. It can seem to come out of thin air, and I want you to begin to say, "Money comes easily to me." Money comes easily to me and to always think, what is the simplest way money can come to me?

But revenue has to do with how you want to get your income.

My favorite way of getting income is passively. What is passive income? One of the common passive incomes is real estate.

There is active income and passive income, and real estate is a great way for to gain passive income. Rental properties are one of my hobbies that I haven't talked with you about. There's also what is called residual income, which means, after you deliver the product or service, the money keeps coming in.

A common way to get residual income is one you may or may not like. A lot of people have strong feelings about this, but multi-level marketing is something where a lot of times, people have residual income for years after they stop the activity.

You have particular revenue streams. If you're working for somebody, earning it, you get a salary.

That's one revenue stream. But when you are building a business, you have to figure out how you want your revenue stream to come in. For instance, when you're coaching and consulting, people pay you for three-month services, for six-month services, four-year services, two-year services. This is what the revenue stream model in consulting is. Think about what type of revenue stream you want. You may decide you want some passive revenue. You may want residual revenue and you want consulting revenue. Or you might want to just stay and have a traditional salary. Also remember, the revenue you don't have to have is hourly, a particular amount per hour.

You can have revenue that comes to you based on the value that you provide. Start thinking about the value that you provide, and how the value that you provide is completely unrelated to the value that anybody else provides. How do you start figuring out what value you are? Well, here's what I tell people, look around at what everybody is charging for whatever you think you're going to do.

Find the person who's charging the most. Then double it. That's a great place to start.

There are many ways you can figure out how to start charging for your services. You can do an hourly rate.

I don't recommend that. I recommend bundling services or doing a package with a lot of services in it that provides a lot of value. There's some things where you may use an hourly rate.

But I'm going to discourage you from thinking about it as hourly activity. What I want you to think about is where you are now and where you want to be, then we'll figure out how we get you there.

It may be a bunch of things together. It may be passive residuals, lump chunks for consulting or coaching, or it may be salary. You can do several at once. Think about it. Now, if you're in an employed position, you can add on a coaching or consulting business with your intellectual property, something you can go home and do in the evenings or on weekends.

Now the "E" in C.A.R. E. is Engaging an excellent team.

The team that works with you is of the utmost importance because, in order for you to be able to have true success, you have to have the right team around you.

Begin to think about the people that you need on your personal and professional team.

Look at your five areas.

You should have at least one person on your team to help you in all those areas. When I say team, I mean people that you hire. They are accountable to you and you are accountable to them. Why hire? Because when you pay, you pay attention. The compensation has to be enough to get your attention and their attention.

Health, finances, career, relationships, spirituality, and personal growth.

If you want to master those areas, the shortcut is the "who." Who is going to help you master all those particular areas? Also note that if there is one of these areas that you are doing poorly in by your assessment, it is likely that you don't have a coach in that area and/or you have not invested time and money in the right way in that area.

Now remember back when you went through your medical training, no one taught you how to master any of those areas. If you say, "Well, yes, they did, they taught you career." They taught you the technical skills, but they didn't teach you how to use it in a business fashion. Also, it is downright rare to come across in your training doctors like me who use our skillset in an out of the box way. Was there a career day in which you were able to meet a clairvoyant eye surgeon or even a doctor who specialized in getting people off of their medications from chronic diseases like diabetes, high blood pressure, or cholesterol issues? Did you meet any practitioners who help people fix their thyroid or other autoimmune diseases? Did you meet a doctor who coaches people how to package and bundle and offer high ticket services? Chances are that I'm the first doctor you come across that has done all things.

Look carefully at those five areas, and assess who you have on your team today. Are they doing whatever they're doing excellently? If you don't have the team put together, start putting together that team. Now let me say something about this. Hire people – do not just pick people's brains, hire people to be on the team.

They're going to give you one hundred percent of what they can give you when you have hired them.

Start with health. Let's think about it. When someone comes to you as a doctor, you give them one hundred percent. You feel obligated and take it as a moral imperative to do what you can to help everyone that comes to you for your professional opinion. If you're saying, "Well, I'm not giving one hundred percent now because I've been burnt out," you're giving the one hundred percent that you can give at that time. You're doing the best you can do at that moment, and that's your hundred percent. I know that's what you're doing.

At the beginning of the book, I told you my story about Mr. I-have-no-letters-behind-my-name. That was my spiritual advisor. He was hired and on my team. I told you about him specifically because where doctors and other licensed professionals tend to get stuck is that they feel they are "qualified" or "trained" to be able to coach and consult. You might even right now want to run off and get a certification in coaching. No! Don't do that. You have all you need right now without one iota of more of anything to be able to coach and consult and deliver remarkable results. If health coaches with nine-month online trainings are guiding health transformations and making $250,000 doing it, you can do even better and make $1 million.

Think about all that.

The next part of engaging an excellent team is to find who's going to help you succeed in your business. You have to find the team that's going to do that, and it may be several people.

You're saying, "Well, how do I find these people and how do I afford it?"

There's a whole industry out there with people who assist and do different things for people. I have a team of virtual assistants, and they each have an area of core genius. For people who become my clients, they get access to my team and I help them find the right team. Because I know that I cannot do everything for my clients, I always bring in other people with different levels of expertise. Think of it like this. If you are an OBGYN, you are going to hand off the baby to the pediatrician because you are the woman expert and they are they baby expert. I do that same thing with my clients. I take care of some things, and I have my team take care of other things.

Marcy's excellent at editing, graphics, and setting up and organizing events. Marcy is special to me because she has been with me for the past six years to support me in building my coaching and consulting business. I've depended on her for so much and learned a lot from her. She has also learned from me about her business and transformed her own health as she followed advice in my materials. She edits and puts together presentations and graphics and, along the way, has picked up enough information to fix some stuff. I'm so proud of her for this. When you are looking at my Instagram or even reading this book, know that Marcy has had a major hand in what you see. Marcy rescues dogs and has even given me advice on how to handle my Artemis and Apollo, my Jagdterriers who are challenging hunting dogs.

Magic happens when you are in flow with your team for all members. Here is what Marcy wrote to me on Slack, as we were editing this section:

"It's a work in progress, for sure. I think what's interesting is how what I've learned from working with you has filtered to my family and friends. You can see the influence in our menu, in what we drink, in how we shop. That's just through osmosis – I'm not preaching or pushing them to read this or do that."

I want you to grasp this because this is about you affecting a far-reaching group of people even when you don't know you are doing it. I know when I hear this that I am on my master path in life.

Michelle is excellent at anything having to do with technical skills, building websites, updating websites, running my InfusionSoft, hooking up my Wufoo forms, getting my Acuity scheduling in order, and anything that has to do with technical stuff. I love chatting with Michelle about her daughter who is a cadet at West Point and her daughter who is a swimmer. I considered going to West Point and was on the swim team in high school. My stroke was butterfly. I admire that she is raising strong, confident women.

Lula is a master at copywriting. She has even helped Hay House authors. I jumped at the opportunity to work with her. When I need somebody to help me with the writing after I've thought through an idea, I say, "Lula help me." She's wordsmiths my stuff from my notes and voice recordings – that's her area of core genius.

My longest running team member is Josh. He's a social media ninja. He has run different types of stuff on all my platforms from one time to another. Josh and I come up with a strategy and he implements it, keeping in mind the latest trends and algorithms.

You might have been thinking at this point that I have twenty-seven hours in my day and ten days in my week and I never go to sleep.

Hair team. Make up team. PR team to get me on TV and in print. Cleaning lady in Pennsylvania, cleaning lady in New York. Dog walker. Dog trainer. Glam Squad that comes to my hotel room for hair and make-up in LA to get me camera ready for filming in the #LoveIsMedicine docuseries.

Whatever I need, I think "Who can do it for me?" rather than "How am I going to do that?" I enlist top performers in whatever I need, and I spend what it takes because I've learned that when I go cheap, it usually means that top work won't be produced, and that means wasting time and having to do it over again and ultimately spending more money than if I simply hire the top person and pay what they ask.

I outsource as much as I possibly can so that I have time and, more importantly, the undivided energy to perform excellently in the areas of my core genius. Number one, helping other practitioners and entrepreneurs get happiness and more money by deciding their best next move and having a plan in all five areas of life. Number two, helping people get transformations in their health to feel awesome by healing their body and spirit, i.e. get their crap together so they can live their purpose.

This is The C.A.R.E. Solution.

It always starts with clarity. In every step, clarity is there.

It always starts with thinking "What is it that I want?" "Is this working in my areas of life purpose and plan?" "Is this in with living my life with gratitude, love, and joy?"

I always ask myself when I'm doing anything, can I do this with gratitude, love, and joy? Am I doing it with gratitude, love, and joy? And if I'm not in a state of gratitude, love, and joy, or at least one of the three while I'm doing an activity, anything, a task, anything, I stop it. I extricate myself from it.

Sometimes it doesn't mean that I feel good about doing everything, every day. Do you know how challenging it is to write a book? Even when you're flowing in the writing, there are parts that feel like pushing the boulder up the hill.

One of the hardest things to do is write a book, and there's parts of it, when you're writing it, that are just things you've got to push through. But I feel love when I'm writing it, and joy when I'm writing it, because of the accomplishment of writing it, yes, but also, I know that when you're picking up and reading this material, I'm helping you, even if I don't know who you are. That brings me joy. Even when I'm editing and putting graphics together and doing things that are not in my core area.

And I'm working with a top coach and team of people doing this, of course. I have to make the time for it. I'm in a state of joy doing it, knowing that I am completely on purpose for my life as I am doing the challenging tasks.

When you are reading this book, I'm in a state of gratitude, because I'm grateful that you kept reading long enough to get to this point in the book.

When you're engaging your team with excellence, think about your attitude and keep it in what we call the "attitude of gratitude."

Are you happy and grateful about engaging with excellence? I'm happy and grateful that there's all these mentors that can help me get those five areas of my life together. I'm happy and grateful that I've found all these wonderful people who have services to offer me, to help me be able to present myself to the world. Do you know what it's like when I'm dictating, and I need editing? I have the perfect woman for that.

This is one of the secrets, the shortcut I learned, and I'm so thankful that I was able to be one of the high performing entrepreneurs that was chosen to be in Dan Sullivan's Strategic Coaching program.

He taught me to always think Who, not how.

I leave you with this.

Clarity. Avatar Attraction. Revenue Streams. Engaging Your Team with Excellence.

The C.A.R.E Solution. Dr. Veronica's C.A.R.E Solution.

Chapter 13

AVOID THESE SUCCESS KILLERS

Up to this point, I have laid out a framework for you to conceptualize what you should do about the rest of your life. Or, at least, to know what your best next move is. I want to make sure that you avoid what I call the "smart doctor syndrome." Now, I'm a smart doctor, too. I know well what we say in our heads. I realize that some of these beliefs hold us back, and I want to keep you from falling into these beliefs. I want to point out where they are, and tell you how to solve them, so that, when you go back and reread this, and you're along this pathway and you hear these things coming up in you, you can make sure to avoid them.

In other words, these are the obstacles that some people never get around, which means they stay stuck in their current situation. That's a bad thing, because when you are confused, burnt out, isolated, cynical, and alone, you are not doing the best you can do for the people that need your help.

Here are some of the things that I hear.

PITFALL NUMBER 1: YOU WISH AND HOPE, RATHER THAN DO

This is the frog in the pot that is coming to a slow boil. Sometimes, though, the frog jumps from the pot right into the fire.

The plan for my life is wishing and hoping.

I talked to an OB-GYN earlier in her career. She was leaving her second impossible job. She was in a position as an employee of the hospital system. She and her partner were expected to do the marketing and building of their own practice. Now mind you, she was working from eighty- to 110-hour weeks, as was her partner. When she went on maternity leave, she was out for ten weeks, unpaid. When she came back, she and her partners were penalized and their bonuses were taken away for lower productivity. They were upset that the practice volume had dropped while she was out. Not only did they penalize her, they penalized her partners, too.

Eventually, after almost five years at this practice, there was a parting of the ways between her partners and the hospital. It sounds like they fired them, basically, because they couldn't get the practice going the way they wanted it to go. The other part of it is that the obstetrician-gynecologist needs ancillary services and other services to be able to do their job correctly. This hospital didn't have some of their services. As doctors do, she was blaming herself when things were going wrong, and thought that she could have done something differently when she was in an impossible situation. What was her answer? Move on to another job where the situation will likely be the same. Hope that this is going to be a little bit better.

With her young child in hand, she moves on, not knowing if it's going to be better, not knowing when she's going to have time to start the next part of her family. Hoping maybe this will just be better if she moved to another place. Hoping and wishing is not going to get you where you want to go. She shared with me her desire for helping in women's health, especially holistically. But the way she was going about it, hoping and wishing without making concrete plans on how she would get there, meant that she was probably reproducing the same position over again. She didn't know that she was doing this. Because the problem within medicine is that we generally don't have mentors who tell us how to create our life the way we want to create it, to the point where, when a person who's a mentor stands right in front of you, you don't even recognize it, because your plan is just to hope and wish that things will be different just because you're in a different institution.

You are a unique person with a unique situation. But your case mirrors a lot of other cases. Let me tell you another story. As I'm writing this, I'm in my integrative medicine fellowship retreat. We did an exercise with Zen Buddhist monks. For one of the questions he asked, everybody answered in the positive. It's interesting, we all walked over to the other side of the room when he said, "How many of you self-identify as not being able to ask for help?"

There are two points to be made here. One, all of us in the room, except for two people, moved to the other side and admitted we weren't able to ask for help. We thought that we were unique. We realize that we weren't unique, and we shared a lot of common characteristics.

Ask for help.

Get help. Realize there are people out there who can help you. Talking about your hopes and wishes is not going to leave you in the pot or have you jump into the fire.

PITFALL NUMBER 2: I'M SMART ENOUGH TO FIGURE THIS OUT ALONE

You're an expert in whatever you're an expert in. Don't you get irritated when your patient comes in, having Googled a few things on the internet, and they feel like they know how to do it just as well as you do. You understand that that's limited thinking, and you tend to get offended by it. I know I do. Now I stay calm about it at this point because I realize that this is what everybody does. I want to go with them.

But on the other side, the little bit that you can research doesn't replace the years of education and experience that other people out there have that can help you.

Remember, being smart is not the same as having the background training, experience, and knowing how to get results quickly.

PITFALL NUMBER 3: I'LL SOLVE MY WHOLE PROBLEM BY GET-TING ANOTHER CERTIFICATION

Breaking Newsflash: You're fine the way you are. You can succeed in anything you want to without getting another certification. Certification is just a piece of paper. It's not going to show you how to use that knowledge to make money. You can make more money and help more people if you start now. That doesn't mean you don't go out and get more education and training if you need or want it. But start whatever you want to do with your life going forward. Now. You already know enough.

"I'll figure out how to do it because I'm smart and I don't need the guidance." A pediatrician I spoke to on the West Coast was planning on going out on her own. She had never ever run a business before in her life. She had been employed her entire career and when offered an opportunity to do coaching, I thought she would jump at it, except she came back with a, "Well, I think I'll just go out there, open the clinic, people will come, a lot of people know me." Guess what? That's not usually the way it works – you can't just hang your shingle; you have to do more than that.

PITFALL NUMBER 4: MY PATIENTS CAN'T AFFORD IT.

Well, I told you that story about my Medicaid patient. I've seen many cases like that in the past. In the present, in fact, I have another patient that walked in and wrote on her form "unemployed." Then, I made a $9000 offer to help her with her problem. She said, "Yes, how can I pay you?" She proceeded to pay, joined the program, and became one of my biggest champions because her problems got resolved. You don't know truly who can or cannot afford it. Please, don't let your money block or limit your thinking. False beliefs block someone else's success.

Offer your products and services to everyone. You may be aspirational to them. They may not take you up on your offer today, but they may in four or five years. I have clients that I talked to in 2015. In 2019, they joined a program.

PITFALL NUMBER 5: I DON'T HAVE TIME IN MY CURRENT PRACTICE OR LIFE.

Busy? This is the way of the world right now. When you ask practically anyone how they're doing, their answer is "Busy."

And with healthcare practitioners, it's busy, busy, and more busy, to the point where they don't have time to take care of themselves. They feel bad about neglecting their family. They're working more hours than they'd like. They want to have a different lifestyle. Yet, they can't make the time to even explore what a different lifestyle would be like. Let me give you the big-time example. I communicate with people all the time by text and Facebook Messenger. I say, "Hey, here's what's going on at the moment, do you have fifteen minutes to chat?" People text back "Sure, I have fifteen minutes to chat." "Okay, let's schedule the time. How about 2 pm ET tomorrow?" And then silence. No answer from them. For weeks sometimes.

I get back to them. Follow up is part of the keys to the king-dom of getting new clients. I know you have to follow up with people, even for years sometimes. "Hey, are you still interested in talking?" No text back for another forever period of time? Next, their insincere apology. "Oh, my God, I'm so sorry, I didn't see this. I've just been so busy. I need to change something because I'm too busy." You're too busy doing what you are doing and say-ing what you don't want to do that you don't make time to listen to a plan for how you could achieve something different in your life. The reschedules and the cancellations? This is your excuse to keep you stuck, the most common form of self-sabotage (or lack of courage to simply say, "No I'm not interested in whatever it is you have to say Dr. Veronica"). Busy is the biggest form of stuck-ness that I see. This is how you mess yourself up. You're going to read this book, you're going to read it slowly, or you might devour it quickly. Then what's going to happen is you're going to get busy, and you're going to do nothing. Weeks will go by and everything will be a distant memory. A year from now, two years from now, maybe even five years from now, you'll still be busy, but busy with what you don't want to do rather than what you do want to do.

We're all busy. Furthermore, we all independently have made choices in life that decide how we spend our time.

You can figure out where to put this time. I started out with the first step of creating White Space to give you the courage and some ideas on how to free up the time in your schedule. The goal of creating your intellectual property is so that you can charge more and work less. Make some time in your schedule to at least get off the ground. You'll realize that making a little bit of time and beginning to offer your products and services will result in more time being available to you in the near future.

PITFALL NUMBER 6: I DON'T HAVE THE MONEY.

You must invest in yourself. You spent those hundreds of thousands on medical training and you aren't getting an adequate return on investment. This is the time you must make a different investment. You have to do it now, or you'll continue to do what isn't working for you.

Let's have a money-finding conversation.

Tap your retirement fund because if you don't, you will never retire because you will not have made enough to retire your debt at the rate you are going.

Next think about your parents, their friends, or their relatives that are distant that you can ask for money from? Can you tap into your retirement fund and borrow against that? Can you do a crowdfunding campaign on GoFundMe? Be creative about how you're going to be able to make the investment in yourself. There are multiple lines of credits available for doctors. Yes, you can. There is money available to you. You just have to go out and ask for it.

Once you implement your program, you'll quickly be able to pay back any funds that you have borrowed. If you ask, there are people out there who will give you money that you don't have to pay back. You'd be surprised that there are benefactors out there for you. All you have to do is ask.

PITFALL NUMBER 7: SHOW ME THE STUDIES THAT THIS WORKS

This is also known as analysis paralysis.

First, I have sprinkled multiple case studies throughout this book, so you can get an idea of how these concepts play out to allow success and transformation in all kinds of areas in people's lives.

There's not a case-control, double-blind, placebo-controlled study on this, or on everything out there. Guess what? It still works. What I say to you is do your study as you go through the steps. Let me know what happens. Make sure you adhere to it exactly the way I told you to. The number one cause of failure is you being noncompliant. That means you don't follow directions and do it exactly the way you're supposed to do it, in the order that it's supposed to be. Second-guessing it and recreating it is what leads to failure.

I talked to a doctor who was referred to me by his friend from way back in med school that he had known for many years. A deeply trusted friend, he asserted. I talked with him, asking, "What's going on? Where are you struggling? He tells me where he's stuck. He can't quite figure out what to do. He knows he's stuck and he also knows that it's about his mindset. He wants to have a virtual practice. He wants to be able to develop a niche. He's following this mindset coach, except he's not, because he stopped doing the work and doesn't know why. This doctor understands that his mindset is blocking him. His answer to get his mindset unstuck? Do some more.

Even after realizing that I could help him with the steps to figure out what was going on with his life and his practice, and help him develop and launch his successful business, it just didn't dawn on him to ask the question of what I could do to help him. He felt he still needed to do more research on a stuck mindset, and get back to following the mindset coach that he had stopped following. He wasn't even clear about what he needed to do this research on. But the answer was for him: more research

PITFALL NUMBER 8: THIS ISN'T REAL SCIENCE, SO I CAN'T TALK ABOUT IT

Well, I didn't go into all the science behind everything that I'm telling you. There is science, and there are studies in different areas on a lot of this stuff. In consciousness, in quantum physics, in business, in marketing. These are all different types of concepts that work across different professions. There are studies on it, just maybe not the type that you're used to. It's real.

PITFALL NUMBER 9: I NEED MY WEBSITE DONE BEFORE I CAN DO ANYTHING

I started out by telling you the story about Mr. I-Have-No-Letter-Behind-My-Name. You don't need a website. You don't necessarily even need business cards. Some of the most successful people out there don't have websites and don't have business cards, yet they're doing fabulous things for people in their business. You don't need a website to get started. You do need to have your URL, and you can simply print up a flyer with information on it, give it out to people, and post it places. You don't need to have a website.

PITFALL NUMBER 10: I DON'T HAVE CONTROL OF INTRODUCING NEW PRODUCTS OR SERVICES

This may be true in your particular situation. But you can put a new product or service into your life outside of your business. This is why I recommend that you start by buying yourself a URL. When you come up with your unique process, one you can offer to people to start your side business, it can become a real business and a full-time business. But I want all to understand the bottom line. It's just like when your patients come in, and you tell them what to do to get success, but they come back with the same problem because they didn't do it exactly as you asked them to do it.

Don't make the same mistake. Don't think, "Well, I'm a smart doctor. I can reinvent the wheel." The wheel is already invented and works great. Do it like it is and make it successful as I've set it up for you. Once you've made it successful in the right way, then you can figure out how to one-up it, and plus-one it, but first, get success on the pathway that I've laid out. This is the time to take responsibility and stop making excuses. Making excuses is your monkey mind.

The Zen Buddhist monks tell us a lonely monkey is a dead monkey. When you're with people in a pack, it can help you. The right group of people, who know enough to help you, will make you succeed. But don't make the mistake. You've heard about the blind leading the blind. A lot of times, in doctors' circles, it can be like the blind leading the blind. Even though we are all so intelligent, we're not savvy enough to realize that the best way to have success is to go for the Who and not How, which is why I told you about engaging the best team possible.

Now in the next chapter, the last chapter of the book, I want to tell you how to get an A-plus plus plus plus, how to graduate with honors, and get the results that you want quickly and easily.

PITFALL NUMBER 11: NOT SETTING AN IMMEDIATE PLAN WITH A TIMELINE

One the biggest things I see with people is that they don't have any clear time goals in their plan, if they even have a plan at all. You haven't sat down and figured out when you want something to happen, or planned out month-by-month what you will do in order to get to a goal. You have to have a clear timeline on how you're going to get there. You can't just drag on forever. The reason why no momentum is developed is because there's no timeline, so if you don't sit for a timeline, it is unlikely you are ever going to get to the end game.

I talked to an internist last year who was suffering in her practice. She just couldn't seem to get the momentum she needed to have enough cash patients to be profitable. She was still taking insurance, and every month was getting worse. When I asked how much longer she was going to keep things the way they are, she answered, "I'm planning on making some changes in about two years." Huh? She was struggling now, she had no idea how she was going to continue to even practice as her expenses were $10,000 a month, and she was only bringing in $7,000-ish. Do you want to guess what was happening in two years? You are right if you said she wanted to pursue some other training, because she felt that would be the secret to getting her income up.

PITFALL NUMBER 12: NO INCOME GOAL

It can be scary to set financial goals, but it's a sure way to measure how you're doing. You have to put the goals out there and keep going for them. People often feel like they're just going to make money without setting a goal in place. It's just going to happen. Well, you have to put the goal out there and keep focused on where you're going. This goes along with setting a timeline. You must always plan how much income, by when, and realistically think about how you're going to get there, and plan how you're going to get there. Include in your plan that, in the beginning, it's going to be more challenging. Then one day, you're going to reach the Tipping Point. Understand that the Tipping Point usually takes a little bit of time. Do some people hit the Tipping Point in a few months? It's rare, so make sure that when you set your goal of how much revenue by when, you start planning twelve to eighteen months, because you're going to have to work, diligently for at least six months to get everything going. You're going to have to work at it consistently.

PITFALL NUMBER 13: WEEDING AND BRAIN PICKING

You've been out there doing a little bit of what you want to do.

It's not quite working the way you think it could work. you see somebody else who has some answers, possibly. What do you do? You say, "Can I pick your brain?" Or you say, "I want your disclaimer form? Can you give me a BA? Can you tell me how to opt out of Medicare? Can you give me advice about x?" Not realizing that everything is part of a system. The one little thing that you're in the weeds about is probably not going to make a big difference in how you do your plan.

This is the area that's also most detrimental. When you pick somebody's brain, you don't get the best of them. Brain-picking is one of those areas where you think you're just going to get that little piece of information for free. What that means is that it's not worth a whole lot. If you want somebody's full attention, you need to make sure that you invest in them. Even though you have another somebody that you think oh, well, I have a coach already. Okay. I've got three coaches right now. If you think there's information that somebody can give you, you shouldn't be calling them and picking their brain. You should be asking, "How can I hire you? How can I have you on my team?" That way, you will get one hundred percent of the information instead of that little piece. Everybody who's out there is offering a whole system, not just one piece of paper that can be talked about in less than an hour.

Chapter 14

THE SHORTCUT TO GETTING AN A+

I know you want to get an A+ in life, not just an A+ on the test. I want you to have an A+ in life too.

I wrote this book, because I've been where you are, I felt miserable. I didn't know where to go. There was nobody there to pick me up. I was alone, I was isolated, I was out of control. I was depressed, I had PTSD and compassion fatigue. Along the way of getting out of this, I learned a few things, which I want you to be able to use as you go forward.

After coaching countless clients through health crises and other clients professionally through business crises and burnouts, my wish for you is that you quickly see which direction is best for you to go next. Part of this is for selfish reasons. If my family gets sick, if I get sick, I'd like there to be some fabulous, compassionate, and free-thinking doctors out there that I can take my family to and that I can go to. The other part of this is that I see a lot of people who need help as I travel to different places. I talk to a lot of different people, lay people out there who are struggling with illnesses and injuries. I tell them what I do and how I work. I've had a lot of them ask me, "Why aren't there more doctors like you?"

You see, there are 7.7 billion people in the world. I cannot take care of them all by myself. I need other doctors like me, to help alleviate the suffering that's going on in the world. In America, the medical system is broken. If someone doesn't stand up, and do it differently, it's going to continue to be broken. People are going to continue to get sicker and sicker and sicker. That means a lot of misery. I believe that every person deserves to have people on their team that can help them. Every patient deserves to be someone's a patient. Every client deserves to be someone's client. That means there needs to be so many more doctors out there who are doing things in a different way. Getting back to their roots, or moving into different areas where they can serve in different ways. I put together this blueprint for you so that you can go out in life and serve again. Let me summarize the steps that you must go through to be able to fulfill your life purpose.

Step One: Take Back Your Time - Plan and Create Your White Space

The purpose of this is so you can clear your schedule and clear your head.

Step Two: Take an Inventory so You Can Take Control

Let's be honest, the purpose of this step is for you to look at the five core areas of your life and identify where you're succeeding and strong, and where you're failing, if you can. There's room for improvement.

Step Three: Find Your Pot of Gold at the End of the Rainbow

The purpose of Step Three is for you to lay out your gifts, your talents, and your passions, outside of your current situation.

Step Four: Get Rid of Head Trash So You Can Figure Things Out

Step Four is so you can clearly see what is holding you back and how to let it go.

Step Five: Claim Your Territory

The purpose of this step is for you to identify your skills of excellence that be can be used to transform your current situation or move in a new direction.

Step Six: Talk It Out

The purpose of this step is so that you know the words and the questions to ask, to lead yourself and, ultimately, your patients and your clients in the right direction with confidence.

Step Seven: Create Your Passion Protocol

The purpose of Step Seven is to define the unique secret sauce for you to use in either your practice or a new situation.

Step Eight: Get More Money Without Working More Hours

The purpose of this step is for you to be able to give yourself a raise by learning how to package, name, and price the products and services of your unique system.

Step Nine: Your C.A.R.E. Solution

The purpose of this step is for you to have an easy framework to do life differently; to take it to the next level so that you're able to stay happy, healthy and wealthy in both your life and your business.

There is a lot of suffering in the world. You see it every day. You have helped people through suffering on a daily basis.

The step that they took is that they decided to come to you and ask for help. Now it is your turn to do the same. This is the way for you to be able to quickly turn around your Titanic. You will hit the rocks if you decide to stay on your current course. You must get a new captain or captains in your life. Reading this book is simply the beginning. Now you have to do something with the material. Nothing in life is achieved alone, so I hope you are able at this point to let go of the rugged individualist complex and realize that there is another way.

Every successful person out there will tell you about the people in their life who were instrumental. It's sexy to thank your parents and a higher being at the podium. Behind the scenes are the countless mentors. Self-made is never self-made. You at least had to admit that it took two people to do something to bring you into being.

I love what I do. I love my profession. I want to see more doctors like me. I do want to hear from you. I want to hear from you with your successes and I want to hear from you when you need help. My desire is for you to be there to help others in a way that you have never done before. My desire is that you get compensated for your true value. I know that you are priceless so let's get the money overflowing in your bank account so that you can help even more people in different ways. Give money to start a clinic. Travel the world and be a role model and blessing to those who are sick.

And I want to have fun with you. My book coach Dr. Angela Lauria talked about the mastermind retreat she is having at Sting's house. Yes, the Sting. I haven't figured out how I'm getting the money or the invitation to go. All I know is that somehow it will happen. It's going to be awesome.

As I plan a retreat for my clients in the south of France, I want you to dream about being there with me in a beautiful place in which we all work on our lives and businesses and go to a higher level. We create together wonderful ideas along with implementation plans.

Life is not meant to be hard. Life is meant to flow and be joyful. It's my desire that you find that happiness (and more money too).

I leave you for now with wishes of success, prosperity, happiness, and health. I send to you the energy of peace, gratitude, love, and joy.

Love,

Dr. Veronica

ACKNOWLEDGMENTS

Thank you to Angela Lauria and The Author Incubator's team for helping me bring this book to print.

THANK YOU

Thank you so much for reading my book.

I know how precious time is for everyone, but especially doctors and other healthcare practitioners who are overscheduled at work and home.

As a token of my appreciation, I would like you to have my Be Honest Assessment. This is the quick-start guide to lead you to make changes in your life. I know how bad you want to change because you stayed until the last word of this book. The first step to real change toward happiness (and making more money, too) is for you to admit that you don't have a path and that you need someone to help you.

So, I am helping you right now. My desire is for you to feel joyful because you are doing your life's purpose.

Use this link to download my Be Honest Assessment.

Spend only ten minutes doing this assessment and then pick one of the five action items to implement immediately – the one that your intuition tells you to implement. Do this one action for twenty-one days and once you have it down, pick another area to implement and so on until you have mastered all five of the action items. Then, you can start over again with another small action in each of the area to implement every three weeks. I created this so that you can succeed making meaningful changes in your life, even with the rest of the busyness in your life.

I would love to hear from you about how this book has made a difference in your life and also how the Be Honest Assessment allowed you to take the first steps.

You can email me at Veronica@DrVeronica.com, message me on Facebook or LinkedIn, or send a note to me through my website contact form. Yes, you can also call my office at 888-886-1216.

Thank you so very much.

With Gratitude, Love, and Joy

Dr. Veronica Anderson

ABOUT THE AUTHOR

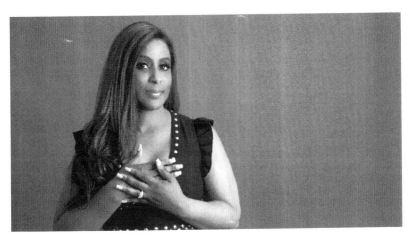

VERONICA ANDERSON, MD, is a burnout-recovery specialist and a physician career make-over coach. Dr. Veronica is the author of three books.

Dr. Veronica began her medical career as an ophthalmologist after graduating from Princeton University and Rutgers Medical School and now has the distinction of being both a licensed physician and a practicing psychic. She is an integrative and intuitive medicine physician, and a certified Functional Medicine Physician. She is also trained in homeopathy through the CEDH. Dr. Veronica has appeared on national television, including CNN and Fox News, and has been a guest on multiple syndicated radio shows.

In her programs, Dr. Veronica uses her gifts and talents to help people with strange, rare, and peculiar health issues who feel like they just haven't gotten proper answers or relief from the traditional healthcare system. Her "Rejuvenation Journey" program guides people to wellness by not only working on the physical aspects of wellness holistically, but also through unlocking and clearing the emotional, spiritual, and energetic triggers of disease, as well as its root causes.

Dr. Veronica's practitioner programs guide doctors on how to use biofield, energy, and intuitive medicine skills in practice. Using her skills as both a business coach and intuitive, she helps doctors recover from burnout, make successful career transitions, and develop practices with their own high-ticket branded services.

Dr. Veronica is a third-degree black belt in tae kwon do and lives in Harlem, New York with her husband and two dogs, Artemis and Apollo.

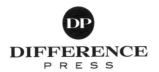

ABOUT DIFFERENCE PRESS

Difference Press is the exclusive publishing arm of The Author Incubator, an educational company for entrepreneurs – including life coaches, healers, consultants, and community leaders – looking for a comprehensive solution to get their books written, published, and promoted. Its founder, Dr. Angela Lauria, has been bringing to life the literary ventures of hundreds of authors-in-transformation since 1994.

A boutique-style self-publishing service for clients of The Author Incubator, Difference Press boasts a fair and easy-to-understand profit structure, low-priced author copies, and author-friendly contract terms. Most importantly, all of our #incubatedauthors maintain ownership of their copyright at all times.

Let's Start a Movement with Your Message

In a market where hundreds of thousands of books are published every year and are never heard from again, The Author Incubator is different. Not only do all Difference Press books reach Amazon bestseller status, but all of our authors are actively changing lives and making a difference.

Since launching in 2013, we've served over 500 authors who came to us with an idea for a book and were able to write it and get it self-published in less than 6 months. In addition, more than 100 of those books were picked up by traditional publishers and are now available in book stores. We do this by selecting the highest quality and highest potential applicants for our future programs.

Our program doesn't only teach you how to write a book – our team of coaches, developmental editors, copy editors, art directors, and marketing experts incubate you from having a book idea to being a published, bestselling author, ensuring that the book you create can actually make a difference in the world. Then we give you the training you need to use your book to make the difference in the world, or to create a business out of serving your readers.

Are You Ready to Make a Difference?

You've seen other people make a difference with a book. Now it's your turn. If you are ready to stop watching and start taking massive action, go to http://theauthorincubator.com/apply/.

"Yes, I'm ready!"

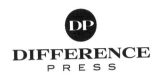

DIFFERENCE PRESS

OTHER BOOKS BY DIFFERENCE PRESS

Going Home: Saying Goodbye with Grace and Joy When You Know Your Time is Short
by Michael G. Giovanni, Jr.

Get Happier, Fitter, and off the Meds Now!: 7-Steps to Improved Health and a Body You Love
by Ell Graniel

Healed: A Divinely Inspired Path to Overcoming Cancer
by Pamela Herzer, M.A.

Live Healthy With Hashimoto's Disease: The Natural Ayurvedic Approach to Managing Your Autoimmune Disorder
by Vikki Hibberd

I Left My Toxic Relationship — Now What?: The Step-By-Step Guide to Starting over and Living on Your Own
by Heather J. Kent

Sign Your First Coaching Client: Steps to Launch Your New Career by Carine Kindinger

Find Your Beloved: Your Guide to Attract True Love by Rosine Kushnick

My Toddler Has Stopped Having so Many Tantrums: The Mother's Guide to Finding Joy in Parenting by Susan Jungermann

In the Eye of a Relationship Storm: Know What to Do in an Abusive Situation by Jackquline Ann

My Clothes Fit Again!: The Overworked Women's Guide to Losing Weight by Sue Seal

How Do I Survive?: 7 Steps to Living After Child Loss by Patricia Sheveland

Your Life Matters: Learn to Write Your Memoir in 8 Easy Steps by Junie Swadron

Medication Detox: How to Live Your Best Health, Simplified by Rachel Reinhart Taylor, M.D.

Keeping Well: An Anti-Cancer Guide to Remain in Remission by Brittany Wisniewski